QUIT SMOKING

The Ultimate Success Formula to Quitting Smoking Now & Forever

(Hypnosis Meditation to Stop Smoking and Eliminate Smoking)

Douglas Lang

Published by John Kembrey

Douglas Lang

All Rights Reserved

Quit Smoking: The Ultimate Success Formula to Quitting Smoking Now & Forever (Hypnosis Meditation to Stop Smoking and Eliminate Smoking)

ISBN 978-1-77485-118-0

All rights reserved. No part of this guide may be reproduced in any form without permission in writing from the publisher except in the case of brief quotations embodied in critical articles or reviews.

Legal & Disclaimer

The information contained in this book is not designed to replace or take the place of any form of medicine or professional medical advice. The information in this book has been provided for educational and entertainment purposes only.

The information contained in this book has been compiled from sources deemed reliable, and it is accurate to the best of the Author's knowledge; however, the Author cannot guarantee its accuracy and validity and cannot be held liable for any errors or omissions. Changes are periodically made to this book. You must consult your doctor or get professional medical advice before using any of the suggested remedies, techniques, or information in this book.

Upon using the information contained in this book, you agree to hold harmless the Author from and against any damages, costs, and expenses, including any legal fees potentially resulting from the application of any of the information provided by this guide. This disclaimer applies to any damages or injury caused by the use and application, whether directly or indirectly, of any advice or information presented, whether for breach of contract, tort, negligence, personal injury, criminal intent, or under any other cause of action.

You agree to accept all risks of using the information presented inside this book. You need to consult a professional medical practitioner in order to ensure you are both able and healthy enough to participate in this program.

Table of Contents

Introduction 1

Chapter 1: Why Do We Smoke? 5

Chapter 2: Effects Of Quitting Smoking 10

Chapter 3: Why Nicotine Is Deadly 19

Chapter 4: Making The Definite Decision To Quit 28

Chapter 5: Controlling Urges Using Nlp 32

Chapter 6: A Look At Nicotine Replacement Therapy 40

Chapter 7: Action Plan 42

Chapter 8: Nicotine Replacement Therapy And Medications 66

Chapter 9: Low-Level Laser Therapy 89

Chapter 10: The Problem With Nicotine Gum, Patches Etc. 95

Chapter 11: Passive Smoking (Its Effect On Women And Children) 97

Chapter 12: Maintaining The New Way Of Life 104

Chapter 13: All Cigarettes Are Similarly Awful 107

Chapter 14: The People Factor 118

Chapter 15: What Happens To The Body When You Quit Smoking? 122

Chapter 16: Quitting Cold Turkey 127

Chapter 17: Lifestyle Changes 132

Chapter 18: Cope With Cravings To Take Cigarette 140

Chapter 19: Organic And Also Holistic Solutions 146

Chapter 20: 10 Things To Stop Doing When You Quit Smoking... 158

Chapter 21: Smoking Does Not Relieve Stress Or Provide Relaxation.. 173

Chapter 22: Five Ways To Quit Smoking......... 182

Conclusion... 190

Introduction

Of all the deaths in the United States alone, one in five of these is caused by smoking. It goes to show that it is the primary cause of death in the US among other preventable causes. Whether its hand rolled cigars or plain cigarettes that you are using, snuffed or chewed, you are in a bucket load of trouble, but it is one you can escape if you try to before everything becomes too late.

Recently, within the past few years, the people's awareness of the negative risks of smoking has increased. Together with the rising trend of healthy living and health consciousness, more and more people have been aware of the threats posed by the unhealthy components in the stuff that they take in their body, like trans-fat, artificial colours and flavours, aspartame and yes, nicotine, which is ever present in cigarettes.

This public awareness started with the results of various pioneer and significant studies in some countries about the negative effects of smoking cigarettes. Of course, people didn't need studies like these to see that smoking is not at all good to one's health, but scientific research has cemented these observations and made these facts, which all people should know and share.

Recently, many steps have been taken to decrease the public's use of cigarettes and even to stop the act of smoking altogether. Governments, for one, have started to impose higher taxes on tobacco products, established a minimum age requirement for cigarette buyers, and started anti-tobacco campaigns which resulted in the banning of tobacco advertisements and strengthening of public awareness through various programs. Consequently, manufacturers have also developed new cigarette products that claim to have less nicotine content. Many new products have also been introduced to the market as safer substitutes to cigarettes, such as nicotine patches, nicotine gum, and electronic cigarettes. However, these substitutes were proven upon further studies to be just as harmful as the products they have tried to replace. Now, more natural ways of quitting smoking is being promoted, shirking the artificial and still nicotine-laden alternatives.

The feat of stopping smoking is, however, a very difficult one; more so if you are planning to do it naturally. This is because cigarette smoking has been part of our lives as one species for many centuries. Tobacco, which is the main component of cigarettes, has always been used hundreds of years ago and throughout history in many countries all over the world.

It was first cultivated and widely used in Central America and Mexico, usually rolled and smoked or plainly chewed, as part of culture and tradition. Tobacco was also used as part of rituals and ceremonies for deities and gods.

With this, it can be said that tobacco has always been an unconquerable foe disguised as a friend to humans for many years. And after all those years, it was just until within the last few decades that we have recognised it for what it is and started to fight back. Unfortunately, it's a hard battle, but not one impossible for us to win.

Though it's tough, there are many ways in which you can stop smoking naturally. And they require more will power, determination, and self-control than any of the other alternative methods out there. Before you start your journey to a nicotine-free lifestyle, it is important to figure out these questions: what, why, and how. What are the negative effects of smoking? Why should you stop smoking? And how do you go about in quitting this unhealthy lifestyle?

This book will help you answer these important questions and more, and will guide you in your quest towards a healthier way of life.

Chapter 1: Why Do We Smoke?

We've all had that day where everything just seems to go wrong and there's nothing you can do to stop it from escalating further down.

Did you stop what you were doing and went outside to take a break?

Did you find a cigarette in your hands as soon as you did that?

That's one of the biggest questions in the world today. Why do we smoke?

We know it's bad for us and there are practically no benefits that you can get from smoking. So why do we still do it?

There are 40 million smokers in the United States alone. That's a lot of people harming themselves knowingly and that number seems to be growing every day.

In order to quit smoking, we must first know why we smoke, the dangers of smoking and the different methods how we can stop smoking.

First off, smoking addiction was not considered as a serious threat in the past. People thought that smoking was a harmless social activity that didn't pose any danger to anyone at all.

That mentality changed when smoking related diseases started piling up and the death toll start to increase.

And here we are now trying to find out how to cure ourselves of this addiction that seems to have a really tight grip on us.

There are many speculations as to the reason why we smoke but it all seems to point to the pleasure centers in our brain. This is basically the same portion of our brain that is attributed to addiction. So in effect, smoking truly is an addiction.

Now what we often see is just the external face of smoking. But what about what happens internally? In the past, people just believed that smoke just goes into our lungs and then we just exhale it when we light up a cigarette. With the help of current technology, further studies have been made and there is a cycle that happens when we smoke.

Take note: since this is a cycle, the first process in the sequence is interchangeable with the next.

1. We light up a cigarette and proceed to inhale the nicotine into our bodies

2. The brain then releases Dopamine into our body activating our pleasure centers

3. Over time, the body experiences a decrease in the level of nicotine in the blood supply which then

4. Activates the brain to create a new craving for nicotine which results to going back to step one which is lighting up a new cigarette or taking another puff.

And this is also the reason why smoking is so hard to remove from our lives!

But just because it's hard to remove doesn't mean it can't be taken out. Don't make it an excuse to continue smoking.

Now that you know why we smoke, it's time to get on to the reasons why we should stop smoking!

Chapter 2: Effects Of Quitting Smoking

Psychological effects of quitting smoking

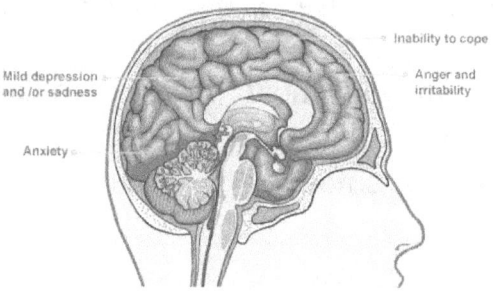

How the Body Responds When You Quit Smoking

The above are the blanket benefits of quitting cigarettes; however, it is interesting to have a step by step analysis of how a smoker's body responds to quitting smoking.

To offer an even better perspective of the gains you will get when you quit smoking, we shall look at the immediate and long-term effects quitting smoking provides.

Just after 20 minutes of cessation of smoking your body begins to undergo changes that will be the foundation of all other benefits. The heart rate begins to decrease approaching normal levels. This goes along with a lower heart rate as well.

As you get past two hours without a cigarette, the changes become even more significant. Heart rate and blood pressure will be closely approaching normal levels. Even better, circulation will have increased, and blood flow to extremities will be improving. You can expect your toes and fingers to feel warmer. However, the withdrawal symptoms of nicotine will have set in and you can expect intense cravings, anxiety, increased appetite and trouble sleeping among others. These are just the early withdrawal symptoms.

Twelve hours in without a cigarette brings about the recovery of oxygen levels in your blood. Smoking cigarettes leads to the production of carbon monoxide. It is important to note that carbon monoxide easily bonds with blood cells as compared to oxygen. When carbon monoxide levels are high enough, they can be toxic to the body. When you go twelve hours without smoking, the carbon monoxide levels in your blood start reducing and oxygen levels pick up. This marks the return of the levels to normal.

One of the serious health effects of cigarette smoking is the high risk of heart attack. Cigarette smokers usually have a 70% higher risk of heart attacks as compared to non-smokers. However, it is important to note that this is one of the reversible effects of smoking. Twenty four hours after you have been free of cigarette smoking, your circulatory system is on its way to recovery and the risk of heart attack though still there is continuously decreasing.

It is amazing how the body just picks up and starts rebuilding even after years of abuse through cigarette smoking. Smokers usually have a reduced sense of smell and taste as well. This numbing is usually not very noticeable, given its gradual nature. However, after just forty eight hours of you quit smoking, a noticeable improvement in taste and smell is experienced. The damaged nerve endings begin to regrow steadily breathing life to your taste buds again.

Three days in and the benefits of quitting smoking are rolling in continuously, however so are the withdrawal symptoms. At around this time, the nicotine in your system will have drain out. Since your body had been used to coping with nicotine, its absence spell a struggle. Cravings will have peaked, physical discomfort in the form of headaches and nausea will also set in at this time. This is usually attesting time and it is best to have a way of coping. Try and get your mind to enjoy other things. This is a great time to reward yourself for the trouble you are experiencing, just not with a cigarette!

A couple of weeks in and the fruits of your labor are accumulating. Your body will have recovered in a large way; withdrawal symptoms will be reduced and most probably at their lowest point and you will be feeling better. Your lungs will be a lot clearer and circulation will have drastically improved. You can engage in physically demanding tasks such as running without struggling with your breath.

The regenerative process of the body continues on and after about nine months you can expect some significant benefits. For one, withdrawal symptoms will have run their course and will be completely done with. Your lungs, ground zero for the effects of smoking will have begun healing. One of the effects of smoking is to neutralize the proper functioning of cilia. Cilia are to the tiny hair-like parts on the inner side of the wind pipe that drag mucus out of the lungs. They help reduce the risk of infection. They regenerate and regain full functionality in months of quitting cigarettes and reduce the risk of infection normally attributed to smokers. You can now enjoy fewer sick days.

A year in, and you will have a lot to celebrate. Over the entire time your heart has been repairing itself, and after a year without smoking you will be able to claim a lower risk of heart attack. To be specific, at this point, the risk of a heart attack is lowered by half compared to current smokers.

Smoking is associated with narrowing blood vessels which resultantly leads to an elevated risk of stroke. This is especially so due to the higher concentration of carbon monoxide as well as other toxins in cigarettes. After five to fifteen years, blood vessels will have repaired themselves to their normal size and reduced the risk of stroke to that of a normal person.

The most common risk when it comes to smoking is the risk of suffering from a variety of cancers, among them lung cancer. It is interesting to note that without smoking, lung cancer would be a rare form of cancer. Over 90% of lung cancer cases are found in smokers. After ten years the risk of suffering from lung cancer decreases by half compared to the risk in regular smokers. The risk of other cancers such as throat, mouth and stomach cancer caused by smoking also reduces.

The fifteen year mark is the most significant when it comes to the reduction of contracting any heart related conditions in the heart. The risk of developing anginas, arrhythmias, coronary diseases and heart infections will have decreased substantially leaving you in better health. At this point, ex-smokers will also have the same risk of having a heart attack as someone who has never smoked.

According to research findings, non-smokers live almost fifteen years longer than smokers. This means that every year you go without smoking, you add more time to your life. Ex-smokers who quit before that age of thirty five are thought to extend their lives by around five to ten years while those over sixty may extend their lives by around three years. This proves that, there is always something to look forward to when you decide to quit and that decision can be taken at any point in life. This is the long term benefit of quitting cigarette smoking.

Chapter 3: Why Nicotine Is Deadly

Nicotine is a very powerful alkaloid found in tobacco that causes cigarette smokers to become addicted, and it's even more powerful than morphine. Let me share a simple statistic:

Of those who try to quit this deadly addiction, only about four to seven percent are successful.

It is not easy!

Cigarettes are the best way to have this nicotine delivered to our body.

When lit, the nicotine in tobacco vaporizes, and enters our system in vapour form and also as tar droplets which are part of cigarette smoke. The lungs and the mucus membrane in the nose and mouth absorb it into our system. Once inside, the nicotine increases the production of adrenaline. The adrenaline "rush" increases the blood pressure, heart rate, and respiration. That is what results in the temporary relative euphoria.

The following neurotransmitters, when manipulated by nicotine, produce some unique effects in our mind and body:

Dopamine gives pleasure and suppresses appetite.

Norepinephrine arouses you and suppresses appetite.

Acetylcholine arouses you and enhances cognition

Vasopressin helps temporary memory improvement

Serotonin helps in mood control and suppresses appetite.

Beta-endorphin reduces anxiety and tension

And this whole process takes a mere 10 seconds!

Since Cigar and pipe smokers do not inhale the smoke into their lungs directly, the nicotine is absorbed indirectly through the mucous membranes in the mouth and nose, thus initially muting the drug's effect. This is no less deadly. These people tend to suffer more from oral and laryngeal cancer.

A smoker typically inhales 1 or 2 milligrams of nicotine with each cigarette, taking 10 puffs over an average 5-minute period. The smoke sends hits of nicotine to the brain.

After an hour or two, as the effect wears down, nicotine withdrawal will happen till you smoke another one. And it continues like a vicious circle.

Make a note, that in order to break this circle, the only way is to abstain from cigarettes till the time you don't miss it. With time, it definitely gives you a kick to be able to live a healthier life. You should have the patience to abstain till the time you do stop wanting to smoke anymore. Even before you start, you need to have enough motivation and determination to abstain for a very long time. That is the whole trick.

Benefits of quitting smoking

To have a rough idea about how fast you recover, the following will help.

Within 20 minutes after your last smoke, your heart rate and blood pressure drop.

Within 12 hours the carbon monoxide level in your blood drops to normal.

Within 2-12 weeks, your circulation and your lung function improves.

Within 1-9 months, you get rid of coughing and shortness of breath decrease.

Within 1 year, y0ur risk of coronary heart disease is half that of a smoker.

Within 5 years, risk of stroke is reduced to that of a non smoker

Within 10 years, your risk of lung cancer is half that of a smoker and your risk of cancer of the mouth, throat, oesophagus, bladder, cervix, and pancreas decreases.

Within 15 years, the risk of coronary heart disease equals that of a non-smoker's.

At the end of the day, what actually matters is the way you feel. Within a year after leaving, you would find yourself much energised. Physically you would feel much more energetic and mentally very calm (cigarettes excite you, make your mind work overtime and increase the intensity of your feelings). The glow of health will be back. It is as if you have grown younger by 10 years.

The best part is that you can have the joy of physical effort back in life. Quitting cigarettes will definitely make you a much fitter person! Life will be less of drudgery and more of joy.

The stages of quitting

There are five stages to quitting smoking, or for that matter, any addiction. Understanding these stages is very useful for quitters as that helps them determine what action or kind of action they should take. It also helps quitters know what to expect. The stages are:

Pre contemplation: This is called 'denial' in medical jargon. In this stage the smoker is not yet aware of the drawbacks of smoking and/or, doesn't want to do anything about it. The patient 'denies' that he/she needs to quit. Wondering which stage you are in? You are reading this book and that means you want to quit and that means you are in the contemplation stage.

Contemplation: In this stage, smokers are aware of the consequences and want to quit. People in this stage are generally weighing the pros and cons of quitting. If you want to quit, but have not taken any action about it so far, you are possibly in this phase.

Preparation/Determination: In this stage, a smoker has already made a commitment to quit and is trying to strategise on how to quit. This is an important stage. Quite often, people try to straightaway move to the action stage from contemplation. These people mostly fail. It is just like starting a battle without a plan.

Action/Willpower: This is when a quitter actively starts taking steps to quit. People are in the actual process of abstaining and this requires a lot of willpower, because this is when the chances of relapses (smoking again) are the most. This stage usually lasts about 6 Months and may vary individually

Maintenance: Maintenance is all about successfully avoiding a relapse or the temptation to return. This takes a lot of planning, determination and smart thinking.

If you have noticed something, since you are reading this, you automatically are in the contemplation stage at least or possibly in the Preparation/Determination stage as well. As people say, "you are halfway done when you understand that a problem exists". It is simple. Acknowledging a problem brings you a lot closer solving it. You can hope to get rid of it now. Here is how.

Chapter 4: Making The Definite Decision To Quit

The first step to breaking free is to make the definite decision to quit! Be decisive, be determined, be committed. Being decisive in what you want is what separates the ones that succeed from those that give up. Don't say "I am trying to quit smoking", instead say "I AM quitting smoking" or maybe even better "I AM quitting smoking for good".

See, by saying you are "trying", all you are really doing is leaving the option on the table to just give up, to just walk away whenever it gets difficult. Is that the kind of person you want to be? A person that runs every time it gets difficult. Everything that you said is important to you, goes right outside the window and is obviously not that important to you. However, the truth is that you are tired of it and you know it! We like to leave escape routes open so when it feels like it gets too difficult we can simply forget about everything we truly want and just run. These moments of stress, however, are simply the experience of a "fight or flight response". We start to feel uncomfortable and automatically seek a sense of comfort. But smoking is not an option, what do we do then? You relax because the feeling is going to pass.

Scientists have found that will-power is a resource and resources are in essence finite. This is not supposed to discourage you, but we have to thoroughly understand this and utilize this knowledge to build a strategy. We will come up with a precise game-plan. You will have the tools to beat this monster. However, understand that yes it can feel difficult at times. People will be smoking around you, there will be times where you are just stressed out and you think it would be ok to just smoke "one" real quick, you will be possibly drinking alcohol in a bar where you are letting lose and might not have as much control over yourself, but in the end, you made the decision because you were sick of it and now you have to walk the walk.

I want you to understand that the whole process is essentially as simple as that:

1) Know clearly what you want.

2) Make the decision.

3) Do it.

It is funny in a way how this concept is pretty much the basis for all success. As you can see, there is no "do it but if it gets too hard..." clause. Understand that there is no "Plan B", there is no escape clause, there is no exit strategy. You make the decision, period. Done.

Chapter 5: Controlling Urges Using Nlp

Neuro Linguistic Programming (NLP) is a set of techniques designed to achieve excellence. They were developed by Richard Bandler and John Grinder in the 1970s and further popularized by Anthony Robbins in his best-selling book Unlimited Power released in 1987. The NLP techniques to control urges described in Unlimited Power have been used by millions of people to effectively control their urges. Here are two powerful NLP techniques you can use to quit smoking. The first technique is called the swish pattern. The second technique is collapsing anchors.

Here's how you do the swish pattern:

1>Identify the trigger image that appears before your urge to smoke. For example, it could be the sight of a pack of cigarettes.

2>Select the replacement image. For example, it could be a healthy you—a nonsmoker six months later.

3>Place a tiny version of the replacement image somewhere on the trigger image and

4>Instantly have the replacement image get bigger and clearer as the trigger image disappears behind it.

5>Take a short break, e.g., look around for a few seconds, and

Then repeat steps 3 through 5 for three rounds. Before you start the swish pattern, measure the strength of your urge. After doing the swish pattern for about three rounds, you should notice that your urge decreases dramatically. This technique allows for many variations, for example, you can swap the images in steps 3 and 4 in different ways.

In the following YouTube video, blogger Tim Brownson shows how the swish technique helps to control cigarette urges.

https://www.youtube.com/watch?v=YtijzExSnrw

This second YouTube video shows a very young Anthony Robbins describing how he used the swish pattern to curb the urge to bite his fingernails.

https://www.youtube.com/watch?v=jPu5cXaTZOw

After you have learned the pattern, one round takes roughly twenty seconds. So within approximately a minute, you should see your urge drop from 10 out of 10 to below 3. It's an amazing feeling of empowerment the first time you experience your urge drop off significantly using a mind technique, such as the swish pattern. Through your own actions, you have become the master of your urges. People who have not been exposed to these techniques really struggle. They are anxious and have that nervous feeling thinking that this time they might succumb to the urge, but by doing the swish pattern or any of the other techniques described in the following pages, you get that incredible feeling of confidence. You realize that through conscious and deliberate action you can master your urges.

Here's an example of how the swish pattern would be used in dealing with automatic triggers. As soon as you wake up, you take the negative image of the automatic trigger. For example, it could be the sight of a coffee mug. Then you take a positive image, for example, you as a healthy nonsmoker six months in the future. Then do the swish pattern using these two images. After a few rounds, you will notice that once you go the kitchen and see the coffee mug the automatic trigger will be nonexistent or at least dissipated.

The second NLP technique for controlling urges is collapsing anchors. Anchoring is simply developing a physical trigger for a useful emotion. We can set off the anchor to get the useful emotion back whenever we want to. To set up a positive anchor, we just revisit a past memory and set up a small physical action that you can do anytime that associates with that past memory. The positive memory could be sometime in the past where you resisted an urge in a very calm way. It could also be the memory of feeling very relaxed and tension free at a vacation spot. Step into the memory to intensify it, and anchor it by doing a physical action, such as placing your hand on the lap. Once you have set up the positive anchor, anytime we want to get back to the positive state, we just do the physical action.

To collapse two anchors, here's what we do:

1>Identify a positive emotion from your past and set off the anchor. For example, the memory could be feeling relaxed and sitting on a beach and you have anchored it by placing your hand on the right lap.

2>Next, think of the trigger urge. For example, it could be the sight of a pack of cigarettes. Anchor it on another part of the body, for example, by placing your left hand on your left lap.

3>Fire both anchors simultaneously. You would place both hands on your lap simultaneously. The effect of the contrasting anchors together is mildly confusing. You just hold the anchors until the confusion clears.

4>Slowly lift the anchor of the unwanted state followed a few seconds later by the anchor for the positive resource.

Within just a short time, you should see your urge drop significantly.

In the following YouTube video, Vicky Dross, an NLP trainer, explains collapsing anchors and how they help in controlling a negative emotional state.

https://www.youtube.com/watch?v=gVPeU2Y2YyE

In the following video, David Shepard, an NLP trainer, demonstrates collapsing anchors.

https://www.youtube.com/watch?v=wO6vGyQLuFo

Collapsing anchors and the swish pattern are the two most commonly used NLP techniques for controlling urges. They can be learned within half an hour, and one round of the technique takes less than a minute. They are a very quick and easy way to control your urges.

Chapter 6: A Look At Nicotine Replacement Therapy

This is a tricky therapy but works for smokers. A nicotine type substitute like nicotine patch is used to replace cigarettes. Small doses of nicotine are given to the body to mitigate the effect of withdrawal but this is done without the intake of the poisonous gases found in the cigarette. One going thing about this therapy is that it helps to break the psychological addiction which will help smokers learn a new way of life

Other Alternative Therapies

Non Nicotine Medication: The difference is that it helps you stop cravings without using nicotine. Examples of this medication include Chantix and Zybian

Acupuncture: This is an old technique that works for smokers wanting to quit the habit. What acupuncture does is to help release the endorphins for body relaxation. It also has a way of managing the withdrawal symptoms associated with smoking

What of Motivational Therapies? They indeed work. Check for materials, resource materials like self help books that are well equipped with guides that help you quit smoking. In fact, some smokers have reported that they found motivation to quit smoking after calculating how much they have to save if they quit smoking.

What If You Relapse or Slip?

The truth is that most people will fail at the first attempt to quit smoking but it is important to avoid seeing it as a failure. You can still learn from the failure and get back to another attempt again. The most important thing is to understand why you have this setback and make amends. Do not give up the quest to quit smoking, motivate yourself and believe you will join millions of people all over the world who have overcome this burden.

Chapter 7: Action Plan

Choose your day to quit: This will be Day Zero and it is important to choose this day wisely.

As you no doubt know having tried to quit before there is never a good time. There will always be a party, a birthday, an exam a holiday in the not too distant future and this will loom large in your plans when setting a date. However, remember what I said about small chunks. Unless you are a friendless recluse or a monk / nun, and my humblest apologies if this is you, then you have a life so deal with it. Some days will be harder than others, accept this and focus on dealing with each day, one day at a time.

My advice will be to choose a date that gives you the best chance of success. In my case I chose the Easter weekend. Good Friday was my Day One and I chose it knowing I would have four clear days away from the routine of work and the routine of my smoking habit.

I chose this date about a month in advance and I would suggest you do the same. During this month I told everyone, and I mean everyone that this was what I was going to do. This helps. Sure there will always be those annoying fellow smokers who will mock and doubt your will power, the world is full of people who revel in the failure of others, expect it and ask for their earnest support. I bet that a few months down the line they will be asking for your advice and you will be their inspiration.

Previously I mentioned my narrow escape in Mexico a trip that started several years before I decided to quit when I was in the fortunate position of having plenty of cash in the bank having just sold a business. Foolishly, one night in the pub after one too many beers I stated in front of all my friends that I was going to the USA for a year and ride a big motorbike coast-to-coast. Soon the word spread and pretty much everyone I knew was eagerly asking me about my impending road trip. Truth was I was petrified. It had been years since I had ridden a motorbike and frankly talking about something and actually doing it are two completely different things.

A year later I walked into the same pub; lean, tanned, with long hair and a book full of stories about my 12,000 mile motorbike ride across the States and Mexico. The moral of the story: you tell enough people you are going to do something, you better damn well do it! The shame of mass disappointment will add to your chances of long term success.

I digress. Choose your day to quit and make it about a month away so that it is near enough to be imminent and far enough away to prepare. Whatever happens you need to stick to this date, do not waver. In your diary (you remembered to get a diary right?) write the words "I QUIT SMOKING TODAY" in large bold letters across the page you have chosen as your Day Zero.

By now you should have been gradually trying to reduce not only the number of cigarettes you smoke but also the times you smoke them. I did not quit by going from 40 a day to 30 to 20 to 10, it would be marvellous if life were that simple but it really isn't. So without keeping count just try to consciously break a few of the habitual smokes. The morning coffee break, the end of the day puff etc. When you quit you will stop for good and it is these tricky routine smoking times that are key to helping you achieve this aim.

The date is now approaching and just before it does you will have disposed of your lighters, matches, unsmoked cigarettes, butts in ashtrays, ashtrays and cigars for 'special occasions'. Very soon you will be a non-smoker, reborn, the first day of the rest of your life so you will have no further use for any of that stuff. The day before day zero you will have changed your bedclothes, washed your clothes and cleaned the house from top to bottom.

The night before Day One you will have the last cigarette of your life. This will be a ceremonial farewell to an old friend. Make it an important occasion; I chose to do it on my own looking at the stars in my back garden and yes it was emotional. Wherever you do it, make it special, you are saying goodbye to your old friend. Before bed, and after your final cigarette you will take a bath or shower, wash your hair and thoroughly clean your teeth like they've never been cleaned before. A clean new you will emerge tomorrow. Day One cometh!

Wakey, Wakey! A new day dawns, your first day as a nonsmoker.

So far so good! Now I am not going to lie to you or sugar coat it but for most people the first two weeks of quitting are the hardest as this is the time that nicotine and the many other chemicals in smoking will still be in your system and will be trying every devious psychological and physical trick to get you to return to smoking, so be prepared. The good news is that your body has already started to repair itself. In as little as 24 hours of quitting your risk of heart-attack and stroke has already started to reduce - and will continue to do so. But for now we are going to concentrate on getting through today. Remember; everything in small bites.

Craving is linked to routine and we are generally creatures of habit. You get up, have a smoke, morning coffee, have a smoke, drive to the office, have a smoke etc. Wherever possible we are going to change our old routines and habits for new ones to break the chains that link us to smoking, but of course eating and going to work are essential parts of our day so we need to learn how to deal with them rather than avoid them. Remember that craving, although intense, is fleeting, so within reason whenever craving hits turn for your NRT. This will take the edge off those moments and they will pass - small bites again.

If, as suggested, you have chosen day zero carefully then you will have the opportunity to avoid any routines today and hopefully tomorrow too. Most importantly keep yourself busy, keep your mind occupied. This will certainly not prevent you thinking about cigarettes and smoking all the time but time will pass more quickly and this is crucial. Dwelling on your situation will not be at all helpfully at this early stage. Sure, you will be sad and emotional.

Think about my analogy of losing a dear friend or relative. This is where you are at. You said goodbye last night and everything is far too raw at the moment. The grieving process will be an emotional roller coaster that you will want to get off, but you cannot. There will be tears and regrets, perhaps even self-loathing, we all handle grief in different ways but remember one thing, time is a great healer. As the days and weeks pass, as with the grief of a physical loss, you will return to normality, a new normality and hopefully a better one enriched by your experience and new found strength. But for now, day zero, it's perfectly acceptable to be a blubbering wreck!

Eat three meals today. Breakfast, lunch and dinner and at this stage if snacking in between helps then snack away. You will probably feel guilty but at this stage it doesn't matter, if it helps then do it. When cravings hit, use your NRT, that is what it is there for. I also found that physical exercise is important from day one. I'm not talking about running a marathon or climbing a mountain but a gentle stroll around the block will suffice. Although you will initially be unenthusiastic about it, a half hour stroll around the block at lunchtime will work wonders. Do it religiously and you will notice the benefits, I promise.

During these early days and maybe for some time afterwards you may feel as though you have a cold. Aches and pains are commonplace and you often hear that those who have quit complain of the irony that they hadn't had an illness for years until they stopped smoking. Well, strictly speaking the act of quitting can induce these symptoms, after all you are weaning yourself off a highly addictive drug. So if you are feeling rough from day one, don't panic, this is a very common experience.

Today will drag. You will want it to be over with as soon as possible but there will be endless distractions and challenges, that devious drug is clinging on and will capitalise on any moments of weakness but remember, it has gone - deceased, for good. One such moment, and the one that catches people out time and again, is the time for relaxation at the end of the day. If, like me you enjoy an alcoholic beverage to relax at the end of the day then I can assure you your defences will be down. In that moment of self congratulatory pleasure at having cracked the first day your urges to celebrate with a smoke, as illogical as it sounds, will be at their strongest.

Here is my advice, based on my own experience: do not try and quit and drink on the same day or days. The effect of alcohol on your brain is too similar to the effect of nicotine and if you are going to slip, it will be after a drink. As hard as it may be if you absolutely want to do this then do not drink for the first week of quitting. As the days go by you will have good ones and bad ones but historically day four, for whatever reason, can be a bitch! If you can see the week through on your best efforts of will power and NRT then your chances of success are vastly improved.

This is a book on how I quit smoking, not on how I quit drinking (I still enjoy a drink by the way) and doing both together would probably be too much for most mortals to handle. For this reason my suggestion, if you are a drinker, is to wait until the weekend after you quit. For me that meant quitting on a Friday and having my first glass of wine on the following Friday. I mentioned the support of friends. Well, this is especially important at this time.

My suggestion is that you invite a friend or friends over to celebrate your amazing achievement of quitting for a week with a drink or two. Always drink in company and respectfully ask your companions to refrain from smoking if they are smokers. Ask them to support you in every way possible and let them know that this time you are serious about your endeavours, be honest and frank. The more you share your reasons and enthusiasm for quitting the more successful you are likely to be. So, do not drink alone, if you do then there is a chance that in your more 'compliant' state you will falter.

Back to day one. Self satisfied, and rightly so, you retire to bed and before turning out the light you take out your diary and write a big number 1 in the middle of the page for today's date and put a circle around it. By all means write your feelings about the day down also if you feel it would help, I did not and this is my story but if it helps then I do not see any issue with it. I will not lie when I predict you will not sleep like a baby! There is a chemical battle of wills going on inside your brain right now that will leave you restless and irritable. It is normal and it will pass.

Congratulations! Every day and every minute and hour that passes you are distancing yourself from the old you, the smelly smoker, and every day you are purging your body of the chemicals you had become addicted to. You should be so proud of yourself, I know I was. The feeling that differentiated itself from previous attempts, the knowing that this was a rebirth, a Renaissance, a chance to be a new healthier you with a brighter future, the feeling is epic.

I am sounding as though you have cracked it, and in a way you have although the path ahead is rocky so be prepared. Firstly the route to be coming a non smoker, if plotted on a graph, would not be a straight line. It would be a jagged one, with lots of ups and downs, but ultimately more ups than downs. The days that follow day zero will have their many ups and downs, micro and macro scenarios and problems to deal with that present ideal opportunities and excuses to start smoking again.

My way of dealing with these was to split my life into two parallel worlds. Sounds a bit weird I know but it really isn't. Let me explain: Life as a smoker and as a nonsmoker is the same apart from cigarettes. The two worlds are intertwined but not inextricably so. The nonsmoker has exactly the same hurdles in everyday life as the smoker but deals with them without resorting to nicotine a a crutch. How do they do it? Easily because nicotine is not controlling how their brains see the world. A smoker believes that smoking is essential to getting them through life's problems because nicotine is telling the brain this lie to perpetuate it's addiction.

Now, imagine you could separate your life: the nonsmoker side of you will continue to deal with everything that life throws their way in the way all nonsmokers do, the smoker side of you smokes because nicotine tells him to, he is addicted. The two lives are not mutually bound and as the addiction to nicotine wanes after quitting, you soon find that you really can cope with life, just as everyone else does - or at least tries to and the smoker fades away into the abyss. Nicotine lies to you and by realising that your nonsmoking side no longer buys the lie you can move on with life.

The days that follow the first are often the most difficult, at least they were for me. The bereavement analogy holds true. Some days there is nothing else you think about while others are only triggered by a smell, situation or memory. I vividly remember day four being particularly difficult. I was an emotional wreck and genuinely thought I wouldn't make it through the day. I was popping micro-tabs and Fishermen's Friends as if they were going out of fashion. If I was to waiver then this would have been the day.

I recall working in 'zombie mode' as if I were a robot, devoid of emotion with a temper on a knife edge. Somehow I made it through and it is achieving a goal on these days that makes the difference. If you can slog it on through in the face of absolute temptation and weakness, and remember I am not strong willed, then subsequent days are a breeze - well almost. I recall the absolute relief at writing a big 4 in the diary and collapsing into bed that night. There were other days like this but they became fewer and less intense.

Completing the first week is a milestone. Shout it from the rooftops! Don't wait for it to be raised in conversation but instead raise it yourself, "Hey! Guess what, I have just completed a whole week without smoking, the first time in xxx years!". Involve others in you story and success and it will reinforce your success and likelihood to succeed. Tell people how difficult it has been but how hard you are trying and wanting to succeed and involve and enrol them in your aims.

It isn't a sign of weakness to ask for support and at no time is this more important than the first week. I have mentioned about having a drink and if that is your thing then ask your friends, colleagues or family to raise a glass with you at the end of the week to celebrate. Also, why not treat yourself to something, a reward for being so great.

Remember my motivation, and I think yours too, should be your health. It is often said that there should be some financial incentives foe quitting, and no doubt there are, but for me it was always health. It is easy to scratch out some calculations to show you will have x amount of surplus cash if you quit smoking but somehow that didn't provide the motivation for me. And, in hindsight, if I am better off I have not noticed any significant wealth benefits. It is an unalienable fact that people spend to their means. Extra money in the bank or in your pocket is great but is unquantifiable in daily living as we will always find something else to spend it on, that is just human nature. So my advice is to concentrate on reversing the detrimental health effects of smoking rather than aiming to squirrel the money away for a big reward for your self. Lets face it, money can't buy health.

During the first week and in the following weeks you will be going through nicotine with drawl. As previously mentioned you are likely to feel flu like symptoms, this is normal so anticipate it. It will pass. Make sure you look after yourself as this will be the best way to keep on top of these symptoms. Eat three meals a day, walk or exercise regularly and drink plenty of fluids - preferably water. You will also feel low, this too is normal, and will come in waves. Regularly eating and exercise will help with this side effect but it is an unavoidable consequence of breaking the addiction. For me it was transient and came over me in waves which reduced as time went on.

Something else that really helped both mentally and physically was what is now known as wellness. When I quit it was more about meditating in a quiet place. Today there are numerous guided meditation videos and audio tracks available to help you achieve inner calm and peace. It all sounds a bit new age but I can assure you it really does work. Being able to completely relax and learn how to control your thoughts is a valuable and free tool which you shouldn't overlook.

 I started on day one and still do it to this day, not religiously but as and when I feel I need to unwind. If you can combine this with gentle exercise, something like yoga, then you will start to notice many mental and physical benefits and it will help you become the new healthy person you hope to be post cigarettes. Learn the techniques now and turn to them from day one. They needn't take much time out of your day but I can assure you you will reap the benefits. Just another tool in your armoury.

From my own experience the first three months were the most testing although to a lesser and lesser tent as time wore on. I kept up my daily exercise, only drank in company and then only in moderation and avoided all social situations that may have put me in harms way. I was also taking NRT to a greater or lesser extent throughout this period as and when the need arose. I did not actively wean myself off during this time which I think is important to mention.

Too often you hear people boasting that they are now only on a fraction of the NRT after only a few weeks when in fact I believe you should do this when it is right for you. Why should you beat yourself up for using support when you need it, be that one week or three months after you quit. If it means not smoking cigarettes then you shouldn't feel guilty. Keep them with you and use them when you have to. For me I started finding I didn't need them as often after three months, for you it might be longer or shorter.

By the time you write 90 in your diary you have pretty much cracked it. There will be cravings of course and situations where you yearn for cigarette but these are less powerful and briefer than before. Every week that passes you will be edging that little bit closer to your goal. By this point your physical dependence will be pretty much over but there will be lingering psychological dependency issues which will surface occasionally. Anticipate them and deal with them as they arise.

You are a nonsmoker now but never relax your guard, particularly in situations where you would have previously enjoyed a smoke, be that due to stress, anxiety or perhaps a pleasurable situation. You cannot, and will never be able to have just one cigarette - no matter how drunk or how appropriate the situation seems.

Nicotine is no longer part of your universe, it is dead to you. Just recall the achievement of getting to this point. Just one cigarette has the potential to undo all that hard work, and will possibly trigger the chemical and psychological hold that nicotine had on you. Do you really want to strike through that 90 and start again at 1?

Nicotine is a clever and manipulative drug and will take hold of your life again at any opportunity. Even now, after quitting many years ago, I still occasionally catch a waft of exhaled cigarette smoke and switch straight back to the pleasures of smoking. This is an automatic, if illogical, response. But the techniques I used to initially quit have stood me well over the subsequent years and yes, I still miss smoking on those rare occasions, but I will never go back - and neither will you.

Chapter 8: Nicotine Replacement Therapy And Medications

Nicotine is a drug, which is inhaled from the tobacco in cigarettes. This nicotine becomes immediately absorbed into the bloodstream, which then stimulates the brain. The majority of people that smoke on a regular basis are addicted to nicotine.

Regular smokers that try to give up can find it is particularly challenging, because as the blood levels of nicotine fall, they begin to experience withdrawal symptoms that they feel they can only overcome by lighting up another cigarette. Those that stay strong and avoid that cigarette will find that after the first 24 hours the symptoms will peak and these can then last for as long as a month, depending on the severity of the addiction.

Long gone are the times when there was no help available for those who wanted to stop smoking, however. This, coupled with the advancements that have been made in science and medicine, means that there are a multitude of medications and therapies that are available to ease the withdrawal symptoms make it far easier for smokers to quit, and to stop for good.

NRT - Nicotine replacement therapy

NRT is a way of getting nicotine into the bloodstream without having to actually smoke. There are a number of places that sell nicotine replacement products and these are also available on prescription from a number of doctors or healthcare providers. There are several forms that the replacement can come in such as:

-Nicotine gum

-Nicotine practice

-Tablets

-Sprays

-Inhalers

Regardless of the form of nicotine replacement you choose, they serve as a tool to stop or reduce the actual symptoms of nicotine withdrawal. It is vital to recognize that nicotine replacement products will not simply make the person stop smoking altogether, but serve to alleviate the symptoms. These products need to be used with determination and will power in order to break the habit.

Using nicotine replacement therapy

Prior to using any kind of nicotine replacement therapy you should seek advice from your doctor, healthcare provider, stop smoking clinic, or pharmacist. Once you have discussed the options with them you will need to decide which type of nicotine replacement therapy you both feel would be best suited to you.

Determine the date that you will start your smoke-free journey, start planning your smoke-free journey and nicotine replacement therapy around that date from the beginning. Most people find it most beneficial to either take the NRT in the morning when they wake or at bedtime, as they will be asleep then while the body becomes accustomed to the therapy.

To begin with, you should use your nicotine replacement therapy regularly, making sure that you use the right dosage, determined by your healthcare provider, for 8 to 12 weeks in order for you to get the maximum benefits and have the best long-term chances of quitting forever. During this time though, you will be reducing the nicotine replacement therapy until you have finally stopped. It is important that you never combine nicotine replacement therapies as they can work against each other and result in serious illness. Again, please follow the instructions of your health care provider.

To greatly enhance your chances of success with the nicotine replacement, it is a good idea to have some type of support in place. The majority of the replacement therapy products come with a support service advertised on the packaging and it is advisable to take advantage of the support, as this will be a difficult time for you to get through.

Is nicotine replacement therapy effective?

There are a number of results to prove nicotine replacement therapy does increase smoker's chances of giving up. There have been numerous studies into the results that can be achieved by using nicotine replacement therapies. These studies were undertaken by two focus groups of smokers, the first group was administered NRT and the other group took a placebo product. The results concluded that 70% of those taking the nicotine replacement therapy stopped smoking where as only 10% taking the placebo had managed to stop. It is for this reason alone that, for the majority of people wanting to give up smoking, it is recommended that they use nicotine replacement along with counseling and all of the other support and resources available.

Which is best?

Nicotine replacement therapies that are available are all different and it is really down to a personal preference and a health care provider's advice on which product would be best for you. The information below has been provided to give you a snapshot of each treatment, however it is important that you always read the manufacturer's packaging for instructions and that you seek advice and an explanation from your pharmacist, doctor or health care provider.

Nicotine gum

This gum is available in both 2 mg and 4 mg strength. Those that currently smoke 18 cigarettes or more per day they would likely be recommended to start with the stronger 4 mg dose. The maximum dosage would be 15 pieces of gum per day. When nicotine gum is chewed, it releases nicotine and the flavor becomes stronger as the person continues chewing, once the flavor is strong the gum should then be rested between the cheeks to allow the nicotine to be absorbed into the bloodstream. Once the taste fades the user should begin chewing again and repeat the process. Every piece of gum on average should last for up to an hour.

After the first 2 to 3 months you will find that you become less and less dependent on the nicotine gum. In order to help with this you could start by reducing the time that you chew it for, or cut to the gum into smaller pieces. Some users have reported the alternating between a piece of nicotine gum and a piece of sugar free gum is a great way to cut down until you have finally stopped.

The downside to using nicotine gum is that a lot of people do not like having something in their mouth all of the time and others may find that they do not like the taste. Nicotine gum is also not suitable for anyone with dentures.

Nicotine patches

Nicotine patches are discreet and easy-to-use; they simply stick to the skin and release nicotine through the skin into the bloodstream. There are a number of varieties and strengths available including some patches that have been designed to be worn only when you are awake for a total of up to 16 hours and others the last 24 hours. Suggestions have been made that the 24-hour patch can cause disturbances to sleep, however, patches are said to be exceptional in curbing early morning cravings.

The manufacturers of nicotine patches advised that the user gradually reduces the strength and their dependency on the patches, however studies have shown that it is better to stop completely and not gradually.

The disadvantages of nicotine patches are that they constantly deliver a steady source of nicotine and they do not mimic high or low levels of nicotine that are experienced from smoking or chewing nicotine gum. There are also some users that have reported skin irritation that occurs under the patches.

Nicotine inhaler

A nicotine inhaler resembles a cigarette, and is used in a similar way. There is a cartridge that contains nicotine which is inserted into the replica cigarette and the user then inhales as they would a normal cigarette. Generally it is suggested that a maximum of 12 cartridges are used per day for the first two months, then the user gradually decreases the amount over the following months. The nicotine inhaler is particularly good for those that want the familiar hand to mouth action that they have that that smoking provides.

Nicotine nose spray

Nicotine nose spray is absorbed through the nose and into the bloodstream, and closely imitates the quick increase of nicotine that smokers get from a cigarette, which is why this product can be most helpful to relieve cravings. However, about one in every three users of the nicotine nasal spray reported suffering nose or throat irritation, watery eyes, or coughing. The spray has been known to cause sneezing, and this coupled with watery eyes. These side-effects are something to be aware of when considering nicotine nasal spray.

Nicotine mouth spray

Nicotine mouth spray acts in a very similar way to the nasal spray and provides the rapid increase in nicotine levels. One or two sprays can be applied as when the smoke it gets the urge to smoke, however users it should not use more than two sprays at a time, and a maximum of 64 sprays in a 24-hour period. The downside of nicotine mouth spray is that reports show it can trigger irritation in the state nose and throat.

Electronic cigarette

The electronic cigarette has become a world-wide phenomenon. It is a battery-powered vaporizer that mimics a cigarette as it has the same feel as a cigarette, without containing tobacco. Generally, an e-cigarette has a heating element which vaporizes the liquid solution. This liquid is made up of a combination of glycerol, flavoring, and there are nicotine and non-nicotine options (since the e-cigarette can be used both by those trying to quit, and those who are continuing their smoking habit).

Due to the electronic cigarette being a relatively new device, there is still uncertainty with regards to the benefits and risks. However there has been evidence to prove that the use of an e-cigarette does benefit those to stop smoking. There has also been evidence to show that the e-cigarette does not have the addiction properties that are tied in with the traditional cigarette. Apart from these factors both products appear to be similar and with regards to safety the e-cigarette comes up to standard with all other nicotine replacement products.

The missions from an e-cigarette have far fewer toxic components when compared to cigarette smoke and an e-cigarette is far less harmful to users and bystanders. While currently there have not been any serious side-effects reported, there have been less serious effects which include inflammation of the throat and mouth, vomiting, nausea and a cough.

Is it possible to combine different nicotine replacement therapies?

Combining different nicotine replacement therapies would only be really be an option for those that experience particularly bad withdrawal symptoms. Again, please consult your health care provider about this. The most common combination would be the use of the nicotine patch, as this provides a constant level of nicotine in the blood, coupled with gum or spray which would increase the level of nicotine and ease sudden cravings. Statistics show that research has confirmed that this type of combination provides a significant rate of success over the use of just a single product.

Nicotine replacement therapy and diseases

In general getting your nicotine via nicotine replacement therapy is a far safer option than obtaining from cigarettes, as the replacement therapy products do not contain harmful chemicals and toxins that are found in cigarettes. Regardless, you should note the following and take care for any that are applicable:

Pregnancy

Due to nicotine replacement therapy being safer than smoking, its use may be justified in pregnant women. Products that are used intermittently such as the gum or spray more preferable than patches as these minimize the exposure of nicotine to the born child. It is very important to note that the licorice flavored products must be avoided completely.

Breastfeeding

The amount of nicotine that can get into the bloodstream is significant when using nicotine replacement therapy. Those mothers breastfeeding within an hour of either smoking or taking a nicotine replacement therapy will significantly increase the levels of nicotine present in their breast milk.

Prescription only and NRT

Currently there are two prescription only nicotine replacement therapies that have had fantastic reviews; these are Bupropion, which is more commonly known as Zyban, and Varenicline, which is more commonly known as Champix.

Bupropion (Zyban)

Bupropion was originally developed as a treatment for depression, but has since been found to help smokers quit smoking. It alters the level of some of the chemicals that are found in the brain, however it is proved to be an exceptional treatment for the relief of withdrawals symptoms that those quitting smoking may experience.

How effective is Bupropion?

While taking it Bupropion there is no doubt that it will increase the chances of you quitting smoking, and there is conclusive research that shows that the tablet has doubled the amount of smokers have quit.

How to take Bupropion

Smokers are required to take one 150 mg tablet for the first six days, and this is then increased to 1 tablet twice a day with an interval of no less than eight hours between tablets. The smoker typically needs to continue taking these tablets for the following seven weeks.

Side effects from Bupropion

Most of the people that have taken Bupropion have had no side-effects, however as with any medication it is important to read the instructions and leaflet carefully. The most commonly reported side-effects are dry mouth and difficulty sleeping. The more serious side effects which are less common could include:

-Seizure

-Drowsiness

-High blood pressure

Is Bupropion suitable for you?

Anyone that falls into the categories shown below or have medical conditions that are named should not take Bupropion. Including:

-Anyone under the age of 18 years old

-Pregnant or breast feeding mothers

-Anyone who has ever suffered from seizure, epilepsy or any kind of unexplained black outs

-Those who have suffered or are suffering from bulimia or anorexia

-Those that suffer or are sufferers of bipolar or manic depression

-Anyone that is currently following a sharp withdrawal from benzodiazepines or alcohol

-Those with a diagnosed tumor of the brain or spinal cord

For all other individuals it could be that the dose of the Bupropion may need to be recalculated if they have ever experienced any of the following:

-Serious head trauma

-Diabetes regardless of the medication that is being used to treat this

-Those who consume copious amounts of alcohol

-Those suffering with liver or kidney disease

Mixing Bupropion with any other medications can also be a risk, so it is vital that you check with your doctor or health provider before you begin with any form of medication.

Varenicline (Champix)

Varenicline was licensed in 2006, and was designed specifically to help those who smoke to give up forever. The way Varenicline works is that it mimics the effect of nicotine on the body, which means that it does not only reduce the urge to smoke, but will also relieve the withdrawal symptoms. More precisely, this drug works by interfering with the receptors in the brain and partially stimulates the nicotine receptors while also preventing the nicotine from attaching to the receptors, thus preventing the symptoms. This makes it far easier for the smoker to resist temptation and give in to cravings.

Is Varenicline effective?

There is no doubt that Varenicline increases the chances of a smoker quitting and there are studies that have proved that those smokers taking Varenicline double their chances of giving up for good.

How do you take Varenicline?

Varenicline tablets have to be taken for the week before you intend to give up smoking, in order for the dose to build up and the body to become familiar with the medication. The normal dosage is 0.5mg for the first three days, then 0.5mg twice a day for the following 4 days. Then the medication needs to be increased to 1mg twice a day for the following 11 weeks. Each dose needs to be taken with food, thus a pattern of taking the medication with breakfast and dinner is recommended.

The course of Varenicline will usually be prescribed for 12 weeks, and by the end of the complete course the majority of people are then non-smokers.

The side effects of Varenicline

The majority of people that take Varenicline will have no side effects however it is very important as it is with all kinds of medication that the leaflets and instructions are read properly. The most common side effects have been reported as feeling sick, headaches, difficulty sleeping or flatulence. The more serious side effects are far less common but may include:

-Risk of heart problems

- Mood swings

- Drowsiness

Is Varenicline suitable for you?

Anyone that falls into the categories shown below or have medical conditions that are named should not take Varenicline:

- Anyone under the age of 18 years old

- Pregnant or breast feeding mothers

- Those with severe kidney failure

- Anyone that with heart problems

- Those who suffer from depression

Chapter 9: Low-Level Laser Therapy

Low-level laser therapy, also called Cold Laser Therapy, is a relatively new technique in smoking cessation therapy that is already making waves due to its effectiveness.

What is Low-level Laser Therapy?

Low-level laser therapy involves applying low-level light-emitting diodes (LEDS) or laser light to specific body points. It is similar to acupuncture only that this time, instead of needles, the treatment calls for the use of LED or laser light to stimulate acupressure points that help reduce cigarette cravings.

A technician administers this treatment and instead of needles, the technician points cold lasers at targeted acupressure points so that the body releases endorphins. Endorphins are natural chemicals that produce a relaxation effect on the body. With the increased presence of endorphin in the body, the body's detoxifying ability improves and the body can easily get rid of excess nicotine in the body.

Benefits of Low-Level Laser Therapy for Smoking Cessation

This therapy has the following benefits:

1. Low-level laser therapy is usually less painful than acupuncture as no pins and needles are involved. If you hate pins and needles, through low-level laser therapy, you can still explore acupuncture as a solution for smoking cessation.

2. Low-level laser therapy is a relatively new technique that has proven very effective for helping people kick out their smoking addictions. According to a

research conducted by Ann Penmann Organization, the Low-level laser therapy has a 65% success rate. The organization reached this conclusion after administering the treatment to more than 40,000 patients.

3. This therapy is drug-free and risk-free, there are no risks of having a secondary addiction.

4. This is one technique where you as the patient can specifically tell if the therapy is working or not. After a few sessions, you can tell if there are improvements instead of waiting blindly and endlessly for an improvement.

Downsides of the Low-Level Laser Therapy for Smoking Cessation

Like most things, this seemingly perfect technique for smoking cessation also has an unfavorable side.

1.   The issue of FDA approval is still a grey area as this technique is yet to get a complete nod from the FDA.

2.   Low-level laser therapy sessions do not come cheap; you have to pay for sessions with a professional.

3.   Unlike traditional acupuncture for smoking cessation, there are no known DIY or home kits you can use; this might be a little inconvenient for busy people.

How to Use Low-level Laser Therapy for Smoking Cessation

To administer this treatment, you would need the services of a professional. You can start by checking this page.

5: Financial Incentives

Several studies have revealed that you can achieve smoking cessation when money you use money as an incentive since you are more likely to pay attention and quit a habit when cash is involved. Organizations are increasingly using this method to encourage their employees to quit smoking and the results have been impressive.

There are several ways you can use financial incentives to stop smoking:

Place a Bet

This is not gambling: what you need to do is to offer a tangible sum of money to someone you trust. This could be your spouse or your kid or any other person you trust. This person would be required to monitor you and maybe follow you around. Whenever you decide to smoke, you lose the money to them. This method can create a very strong motivation to quit smoking since you would not want to lose your money.

However for this to work, the money must be a sizable enough that you would be unwilling to lose it and the trustee must be available round-the-clock to ensure close monitoring.

The Piggy Bank System

The Piggy bank system is another interesting method that helps you clearly see just how much your smoking habit is costing you so that you can divert the funds to something beneficial and satisfying.

Every time you crave a stick of cigarette, you place an amount equivalent to the cost of a stick of cigarette in your piggy bank. At the end of each week, you open the piggy bank, bring out your money, and spend it on something you find rewarding, something positive.

The financial incentive method is very effective when used in tow with other techniques because it brings the financial consequences of your addiction to the forefront and makes the habit less desirable.

This would be a perfect technique for you if you fall below the average income level and if you have any debts or are struggling with various financial issues.

Chapter 10: The Problem With Nicotine Gum, Patches Etc.

You'll find any number of "stop smoking" aids at the drug store. The obvious ones are nicotine gum, lozenges or patches.

Nicotine-based product all have the same basic and obvious flaw: You may just be exchanging one nicotine addiction for another one.

This seems to be especially true of nicotine gum. Long-term users become as enslaved to the nicotine gum as they were previously enslaved to cigarettes. They may get fewer complaints from the non-smokers around them, but the long-term side effects are pretty grim.

Nicotine gum users sometimes report severe problems with their teeth and jaws from constant chewing. Other problems include hiccups, upset stomach, persistent heartburn, belching, and sore throat. Allergic reactions may include an unexplained rash, hives, or other itching. Want more? How about uexplained swelling of the mouth, lips or throat. More rarely symptoms may include nausea and vomiting, difficulty breathing or swallowing, extreme dizziness, diarrhea, and rapid heartbeat.

To be fair, these side effects are generally experienced with chronic use. Use these products if you think they will help, but always think of them as temporary supplemental strategies at best. They may make some sense if you're only using them the first couple of weeks. Beyond that, you're just swapping habits.

Chapter 11: Passive Smoking (Its Effect On Women And Children)

Smokers around the globe doesn't only hurt themselves but also force their neighbours and their near and dear ones to inhale the poisonous smokes of tobacco with them.

If it helps all the smokers to know and help them quit, even if not for themselves but for their loved near ones that non-smokers who inhale the furious gas of tobacco have increased risk of lung cancer by almost 20%to 30%.

Passive smoking can also cause death among non-smokers.

Second hand tobacco smokes also contains all the harmful chemicals that are cancerous in nature.

Passive smoking is not safe.

Tobacco smokes hangs in mid-air and even tends to move down in a room because tobacco smokes cools easily. hot air rises up and since tobacco smokes are heavier than air so it climbs down.

Chemicals such as ammonia, sulphur and formaldehyde irritate the eyes irritate the eyes nose throat and lungs. All these chemicals are harmful to specially people having respiratory disorders like who have bronchitis asthma. Second hand smokes triggers the coughing problems and worsens their conditions.

A lady who is pregnant and is exposed to second hand smokes during this period can give birth to a baby with low weight and if over exposed to smokes then risks of miscarriage and premature birth or even death in infants can happen.

An infant if exposed to tobacco smokes during the first 18 months after their birth can have a range of respiratory troubles associated with them for life; they may also develop coronary heart diseases.

Second hand smoking can cause levels of antioxidants vitamins in the bloods to be reduced.

A person who is long exposed to passive smoking has the risk of developing atherosclerosis.

Researchers have shown that increased contacts with second hand tobacco smokes increases the chances of nasal sinus, lung cancer and other respiratory diseases.

What can you do to avoid passive smoking?

Make sure that your children are with people who are non-smokers.

Do not take them to places where people generally smoke and you have very less options of getting out from there.

Tell the people if there are smokers in your house, to go and smoke outdoors away from children, including yourself if you are smoking.

Try not smoking inside cars, even if the windows are open, the stink or the odour usually stays.

Try to make your home and the surrounding places smoke free, like the garage, garden etc.

When you go about into quitting smoking, always remember that you are not only hurting and endangering your own self and your life but your near and dear ones are also bearing the brunt of your actions. You are hurting your children, your spouse, even your beloved pets and plants are also grinding with this fatal addiction. All of them are falling in the category of passive smoking. Have you ever stopped to think, that even unknowingly you are making your loved ones very ill. I know you never want to. You work so hard, till late hours, so, that they can have a pleasant life, so that you can buy them all the comforts and luxuries. You can give them all the opportunities they need to make them able and successful, but even unknowingly and unintentionally, you are hurting them, not only physically, but emotionally too.

Now, you may ask how? Well, when you smoke, around them, they constantly fear for your life, as you alone handle all the financial stress, workloads and this bad habit is slowly taking you away from them, into the jaws of uncertainty, that when might their father or their better half fall into the jaws of death because of this habit. You are also exhausting your finances with this addiction, by not only buying death, but also making you and your family's medical expenses go higher. If you have a little son or daughter, then they are getting the inspiration to get addicted from you. They would feel the addiction either to be an action very manly or else, they would associate this habit with maturity and growing up, not knowing the reality.

Researchers suggest that the children who are constantly exposed to such environments are not only tormented physically but they are also more prone to get addicted to this habit or may be to other fatal addictions compared to other children who enjoy an addiction free environment.

Chapter 12: Maintaining The New Way Of Life

After the first couple of weeks you'll find it a lot easier to stay away from your old habit. The nicotine addiction is gone which leaves only the minor habit of having something in our hand.

The 3rdweek is a pretty good time to start doing some exercise. Your lung function should be improved by now and what a better thing to do then some jogging? It's very important that you start living a more active life. In order to maintain and improve your health physical and mental you have to find something that excites you. We all have jobs, some are stressful others not so much but at the end of the day you have to be happy with who you are and what you're doing. I know that you'll be happy for what you've accomplished for the past couple of weeks and that getting to this point was everything else but not easy.

Truth is…if you managed to get past that second week without smoking you're a real hero and you have full control over your mind. You should be proud of what you've accomplished and last but not least, you should help other people too. Use your experience in that manner to give your knowledge. It is proven that we're genetically determined to help each other. Nothing can compare to the feeling of helping out someone and this feeling is the secret energy that we all need to maintain a healthy and happy life.

Don't get me wrong, I'm not expecting you to become philanthropist but having the right attitude towards the people around you will not only lead to a better social status but to a longer life.

I know that most of you would say that it's easier said than done, but think about it...every incredible thing that happened in our life wasn't easy. Fighting for what we want, for how we want to live and finally reaching to our goals...that's the sweetest thing.

Chapter 13: All Cigarettes Are Similarly Awful

Obviously the more cigarettes you smoke the more damage you welcome for yourself. Realizing this would make you incredibly stupid on your part not to perceive the effect of the damage even a solitary puff can cause you. Smoking any number of cigarettes is really destructive; in spite of the fact that the level of mischief goes up with each expanding number of cigarettes.

Your smoking enslavement couldn't care less about the trademark highlights of a specific cigarette. It thinks just about getting the nicotine that your body hungers for. Regardless of whether it originates from a separated or a menthol cigarette, whether you smoke less oftentimes or more the drawn out outcomes are the equivalent. Smoking rots your lungs first and afterward every other piece of your body with each harmful smoke you breathe in.

Intellectually Prepare Yourself to Quit Smoking

There are a ton of examples in life when one has genuine questions of what he is prepared to do. A typical marvel is the point at which a smoker ready to stop his propensity feels that he is a survivor of his conditions and that causes him stress. Finding a fruitful method of stopping smoking is a difficult undertaking however in the event that you can discover a recipe for stopping that works for you, at that point you are probably going to be effective. It is essential to envision that you have effectively stopped smoking before you even beginning. On the off chance that you build up that vision, at that point it will be simpler for you to achieve your objective.

It is significant for you to comprehend that how you see yourself and how you think has an incredibly huge effect on your chances of stopping. Commonly smoking is only an indication of different issues one has. The concealed under lying reasons which force an individual to smoke need to likewise be routed to help the smoker in his recuperation. A portion of these issues might be and include:

Help from pressure

Disposing of fatigue

Attempting to fit into a picture

Attempting to impersonate the gathering he has a place with

Loss of weight

Compulsion

So preceding wanting to stop smoking, it is significant that you investigate the reasons which constrained you to go to smoking. You can supplant smoking with other more beneficial substitutes to deal with your root issue. In such a case, you won't capitulate to the enticement of smoking in that specific circumstance. Since every individual is extraordinary, it is basic that everybody builds up his own specific manners of stopping smoking. For instance, my dad who was an energetic smoker would take a bit of treats each time he wanted to smoke. Albeit present day medication makes the adapting of nicotine withdrawal simpler, my point is you have to locate a substitute or outlet during the span of your recuperation procedure.

There is another planning which you can make intellectually. Quit considering cigarettes to be a wellspring of delight, however as something you wish to dispose of. Each time you get an inclination to smoke advise yourself that each extra puff you take is a moment of your life you will never get back. You should be solid and acknowledge smoking influences your life, however it influences the life of each one of everyone around you. Another beneficial activity is to make a rundown of every single awful thing which won't transpire in the event that you quit smoking. Likewise help yourself to remember the beneficial outcomes of a non-smoking life. Battling the propensity is difficult, yet keeping a day by day "reference sheet" or hanging up signs around your home will assist you with remaining centered. One reason why individuals return to smoking is that they wind up saying "this will be the last one." Obviously, they come back to the propensity. On the off chance that you convey day by day updates that keep you concentrated on your strategic will be bound to remain reliable with your approach.

The progress of stopping smoking includes a couple of stages. As a matter of first importance, distinguish yourself as an individual who doesn't smoke, and revise your conduct likewise. Consider what not smoking would intend to you regarding profiting your life. In the event that you have to change your life plans with respect to how you invest energy at that point do as such. Likewise get some information about which hour of the day do you get yourself generally helpless against surrender to the enticement of having a smoke. Recognize the reasons that propel you to do that during that time. Contemplating these things ahead of time will assist you with doing combating the compulsion to smoke when these circumstances emerge.

Positive reasoning is another factor which will help you a great deal in kicking the propensity. With a positive outlook you can go far in supporting yourself in accomplishing your objectives. On the off chance that you can envision yourself as a non-smoker and feel how great it would be; that by itself will give you a ton of inspiration to stop the propensity. Other than the particular given representations, settle on some unwinding methods too. These will assist you with overcoming your inclinations somewhat as they emerge. They would likewise help you a great deal in de-focusing on yourself. You can do a quest online for unwinding methods and even consider what sort of strategies others who have effectively stopped smoking, have utilized. In light of your way of life, you can choose one, or a blend of numerous techniques that you can us to help you through your recuperation. Additionally attempt to build up a propensity for giving yourself a little treat on consummation of every week when you haven't smoked. A similar way that individuals on slims down have "cheat-days" you should likewise remunerate your positive conduct for not smoking. Despite what might be expected, in the event that you end up slipping go into your propensity, stop and re-center. Try not to rationalize, don't attempt to support it, simply stop, and refocus.

Job of Will Power in Quitting Smoking

The idiom "where there is a will, there is a way" is applicable, particularly in the event that you are attempting to stop smoking. The solid assurance and resolution you display will help you in cruising through the most unpleasant of climate. Cigarettes are exceptionally addictive as we as a whole know, and the more you attempt to stop smoking, the more you'll end up attracted to them. Consider it like this. On the off chance that you've been eating chocolate cake for most of your life and you choose one day that you will never take another cut again – you are going to discover stopping troublesome. Smoking is a propensity you got throughout the years, attempting to leave it surprisingly fast will be hard, yet it isn't outlandish.

In the event that you continually consider how the entirety of your endeavors to stop smoking in the past have fizzled, at that point you rout yourself before you even start. Numerous individuals giggle at the possibility of positive certifications – yet they truly help. Two times every day, plunk down and read off a piece of paper phrases like "Today is one more day that I am nearer to getting my life back. I have chosen to stop smoking for me, yet additionally for the ones I love. I am cheerful, solid, and appreciative that I have the resolution and backing to leave this propensity. Smoking was my decision, and now I am deciding to stop. Cigarettes will never have power over my life again, today I take control".

A great deal of smokers everywhere throughout the world have had the option to dispose of the dependence on nicotine. Have you thought about how they have had the option to dispose of this inconceivable assignment? There is no enchanted equation for this, however there are only a couple of steps which you can take for accomplishing your objective.

To begin with, before you can transform you, you have to alter your perspective. Brain research has a great deal to do with stopping smoking. You have to alter your disposition and feel that not smoking would do you a lot of good. Remember that stopping smoking requires a great deal of work and there will be times when you need a convenient solution. You should be engaged and solid consistently. The psyche brain will consistently attempt to thwart your arrangement by bringing into light invented inconveniences of a non-smoking life, yet that is where you should be solid. Simply center around the positive viewpoints and the existence which you would blessing yourself with on the off chance that you quit the propensity for smoking.

To summarize, it's your assurance and resolve which will go to your guide while you attract up an arrangement to lead a without smoking life. Medication will assist you with the physical desires of puffing ceaselessly, yet to stop the propensity for good, you should be set up to make changes intellectually.

Chapter 14: The People Factor

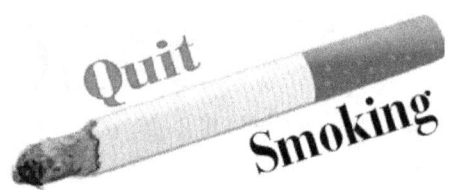

Yes you started smoking alone but if you want to quit, you might need the help of strong willed and helpful people, the truth is it isn't compulsory but it makes it easier after more heads are better than one.

You can't just pick anybody though, you need people who have certain characteristics and I would like to list some here

The person must know he or she CAN'T make you quit but they can offer much needed encouragement and a slight nudge, so nagging or being too forceful isn't allowed, they will need to be versed in helpful encouragement instead.

A busy person you can work with is very preferable because that keeps your mind off the need to use cigarettes, another useful thing is someone who can keep the constant supply of gum ,carrots, mints and other helpful items coming to keep your mouth busy.

You will need someone who is rarely tired of encouraging and would stay with you even if you slip back into the habit which can happen and doesn't mean you are weak

Finally you need a person who will many times put their feet down if there is a trigger around, triggers includes lighters, matches and cigarette packs.

SUPPORT GROUPS

It is great to have just one friend helping you quit but it is far better if you join a support group because statistics reveal that group therapy increase our chances of quitting by 30% and it can be more comforting being in close proximity with people going through the same challenge you are trying to overcome

It is also a huge encouragement to see people around you making progress because you tell yourself if they can do it then I can do it and you don't even have to bother about the price because there is at least one around you especially in your local hospital that is free.

Even though it is free there are still some factors you have to look out for and they are

The group must be led by a certified therapist

There must be brotherly camaraderie there and it must feel like a bunch of friends or you might leave worse than you started.

They must encourage combination therapy, meaning the group must allow you use other forms of treatment like patches.

They shouldn't be short and lack a system that works over time

If you are paying it must not be too high and if they sell pills and supplements that is only available through the program then run like hell because they are probably scam artists

If they promise an easy path to quitting then they maybe fraudulent so back off.

Finally they must have a track record and should be able to point to people they have helped quit.

I should add that even though group therapy can be really potent and helpful, if you are not comfortable with sharing your smoking challenge in a room full of people then you should try and get comfortable first or just stick to the personal touch first.

Chapter 15: What Happens To The Body When You Quit Smoking?

Everyone knows that smoking is not healthy, but do you know what exactly happens in the body when you stop smoking? Your body becomes healthier - from head to toe.

Read here what exactly happens?

20 minutes

As early as 20 minutes after the last cigarette, the blood pressure and pulse begin to drop to a normal level.

8 hours

After 8 hours, the carbon monoxide content in the blood has dropped to a normal level, and the oxygen content has reached normal values.

24 hours

The risk of a heart attack is already minimized after 24 hours.

48 hours

After 48 hours, the sense of smell and taste improves as the nerves are repaired.

2 weeks - 3 months

It takes between 2 weeks and 3 months before it becomes easier to take longer walks. Your burn and lung function can improve up to 30%.

1-9 months

Between the 1st and 9th month, the body begins to have more energy. You cough less and experience less breathlessness. The lungs recover, and the risk of infection decreases.

1 year

If you have been smoke-free for 1 year, the risk of heart disease is halved compared to non-smokers.

5 years

After 5 years without smoking, the mortality rate for lung cancer is halved compared to a smoker. The risk of developing mouth, throat, or esophageal cancer is also halved. The risk of stroke is now on the same level as that of a non-smoker.

Ten years

After 10 years without smoking, the mortality rate for lung cancer is the same as that of a non-smoker.

15 years

Congratulations! 15 years after you quit smoking, the risk of heart disease is now at the non-smoking level.

Chapter 16: Quitting Cold Turkey

This approach helps you fully detox your body of marijuana. Marijuana remains in the system for at least 42 days after the last joint has been smoked. To fully rid the body of its toxic effect and overcome your addiction, you have to set your goal and not smoke up for six weeks altogether. Once the six week period is over, you will have no dependence on marijuana, will not crave it, and can easily avoid it.

Step 1 - Get Rid of Marijuana

Most people, when it comes to quitting, prefer to use up the stash they have. This obviously never works out. When you make up your mind and want to quit marijuana, throw away your entire stash. Dispose it in such a way that you cannot go back and retake it. It may seem like you are wasting money by throwing it away, but think about how much you will be able to save when you stop smoking it. Throw away all your lighters and anything else that has to do with marijuana. It is the hardest and most tempting in the initial days when you cease to smoke. Flush away your stash, throw away the filter papers, etc. Remove the dealer from your contacts so that it is impossible for you to contact him even if you want to.

Step 2 - Get Rid of the Triggers

The desire to smoke up is usually triggered by something once you are a regular user. It could be a movie, music, or a game. So you have to get rid of these triggers so that nothing reminds you of it and nothing makes you want to smoke up. It may seem like going too far but it is very important. If there are no triggers, there is no temptation.

Step 3 - Make Your Decision Known

Let your family and friends know that you are quitting. If things get hard, you will have support. Your friends will make sure that you do not relapse and help you along the way. If they smoke up, they will try to not do so in front of you so that you do not get tempted. If you have friends who are addicts or, are people who you know, will continue to use around you, then its best that you avoid them completely for at least six weeks.

Step 4 - Find Ways to Keep Yourself Busy

You will have to set up a new routine to keep yourself busy. Find new activities and hobbies that keep your mind off the drug. Reading novels that interest you can keep you occupied for hours. Make a schedule, write it down, and make sure that you have something to do throughout the day, for each hour. It can be as simple as an hour dedicated to sitting or hanging out with family. Just make sure that it does not include something that leaves you alone with yourself with nothing to do.

Step 5 - Prepare for the Withdrawal Symptoms

The first thing you are likely to notice, feel, and experience will be a withdrawal symptom. You can deal with the withdrawal symptoms better if you are mentally prepared for them. Do not let them weigh you down. Be ready and take a proactive approach to dealing with the symptoms. Tell the people around you so they can be more supportive and understanding. Others can help you better if they know what is going on. You may lose your appetite but it is important to eat. Include fruits in your diet. One of the withdrawal symptoms is decreased energy. Fruits are packed with energy and are good sources of vitamins, minerals, and nutrients.

You can also join a gym. Replace smoking up with working out. Working out improves the blood circulation. It becomes difficult to fall asleep when you quit marijuana, but working out will make you tired and can aid in sleeping. You will begin to notice changes in your body, like increased body temperature. Keep your mind off these things by engaging in other physical activities like swimming. Talk to your friends on phone or hangout with them, it will be a good distraction.

Step 6 - Avoid Marijuana

Once the 42 days are over and marijuana is out of your system, it is time for you to move on to a healthier life, but also remember to avoid marijuana.

If someone offers you marijuana, say no.

If you see your friends smoking marijuana, leave the scene.

If you have an urge to smoke up, do something else instead. Keep mints or chewing gum with you.

The worst symptoms are over after 12 days. After that, it becomes really easy. All you have to do is avoid marijuana and not smoke up again.

Chapter 17: Lifestyle Changes

Living a healthy lifestyle once you quit smoking is important to make your body fully capable of coping with the symptoms of nicotine withdrawal. It also shows your commitment, not just in quitting a harmful habit, but in adopting healthier habits and embracing life.

Diet, in particular, will play a crucial role in your fight against cigarette smoking. Some quitters experience drastic drop in weight due to loss of appetite. In most cases though, quitters experience uncontrollable weight gain weeks or months after quitting as their metabolism temporarily slows down in the absence of nicotine. This is not a permanent physiological change, but it can leave you with lasting consequences if you take your health for granted.

Furthermore, there are a lot of food that aggravate your urges for smoking, so you also have to pick what you eat carefully. Many of these food will be discussed shortly, but you should remember that food selection is only one half of your weight and health concerns. The other half belongs to physical activity, which includes regular exercise.

Food and Diets

Try different distinctive flavors

Your taste buds will definitely miss the taste of cigarette and smoke in your mouth. Whenever you feel like your tongue is craving for the familiar tastes, feed it with different distinctive flavors instead. You can start by snacking on different citrus fruits and fruit blends, assorted-flavored candies, and palatably bitter dark chocolates. Eating anything that tastes close to the flavors of your former cigarette brand is not a good idea.

Eat to a satisfactorily full stomach

Eating too much makes you want to get rid of the aftertaste and discomfort in your stomach. Eating too little makes you want to satisfy your hunger with something else. In both cases, you end up resorting to cigarette smoking, or at least remind you of that. That is not a good way to start kicking the bad habit.

Eating just enough to satisfy your hunger does not only prevent you from feeling the unnecessary craving; it also helps your body produce a hunger hormone called leptin, the one in charge in suppressing appetite and craving. In effect, it also suppresses your craving for cigarette. Eating the right amount in every meal, every day, is already a big step forward when you are trying to quit smoking for good.

Have something to chew, bite, or hold in your mouth when needed

Sometimes, the urge to smoke does not really come from the craving for the taste; it comes from the habit of getting something in your mouth. You can fight the urge by chewing a gum (not a nicotine gum), sugar-free candy, candy stick or lollipop. Sugar-free or low-sugar gummy candies can also help a lot since the chewing motion already reduces the urge by 50%. At home, always have vegetable sticks prepared in your fridge. You can also eat breadsticks for snack.

If you just have the urge but you do not want to eat anything, just have a toothpick between your teeth, or a cinnamon stick if you want something with flavor. Either one works just fine.

Stay away from addicting food

Getting addicted on certain food will only remind you of your former addictions. Stay away from coffees, teas, any alcoholic beverages, and sugary food as much as possible. Any caffeinated drink is also a bad choice. Delicatessen, barbecue, and any food with a smoky taste should also be scratched out of your diet.

Not all vegetables are also good for you at this point. Corn, horseradish, and peas are said to stimulate craving for cigarettes.

Physical Activities

Find a hobby that you can enjoy

An old bad habit has to be replaced with a new good one. Finding a hobby that you can be passionate about can eat up the time you originally used up on smoking, and spent on something more worthwhile and safe. A new hobby can also take away your attention from all the temptations to go back into being a smoker.

Furthermore, according to studies, people who have enjoyable hobbies have higher amounts of feel-good hormones in their bodies. That makes them more resistant to the effects of increased stress hormone, so they are bound to feel fewer mental, emotional, and physical changes after quitting.

Finding a new source of happiness and satisfaction is also important as nicotine made you feel and think that smoking was the ultimate provider of all of that. You do not have to rely on it if you can find a really compelling replacement.

Exercise for 30 minutes a day

People who exercise regularly are twice as likely to succeed in kicking the old habit for good. Experts explain that exercising is practical and scientific at the same time.

First, exercising prevents you from being idle, which is the time when you are more vulnerable to the temptations and urges of smoking. The time you spend on exercising is the time you take away from smoking.

Second, it allows you to fight the symptoms of nicotine withdrawal, as activity allows your muscles to release tension, thereby reducing risk of muscle spasm. The improved blood circulation also reduces the risk of suffering from headaches. In general, the level of the hormone endorphin—a natural pain reliever—increases when you exercise, which makes you more resistant to the pain and discomfort caused by nicotine withdrawal.

Third, exercising lowers the production of cortisol, which means you get to experience lower stress. This also reduces the urge to smoke drastically.

Lastly, exercising boosts the production of other feel-good hormones in your body. This can help you feel and think more positively while fighting the urge to smoke.

Chapter 18: Cope With Cravings To Take Cigarette

When you decide to avoid those things that will always make you to smoke, it will help you in reducing how you indulge in the act; nevertheless, all those things that will make you to always smoke will not be wiped out totally. It will interest you to know that all those things that always push you to smoke do not last up to 15 minutes; this can be about 4 or 8 minutes. When you've the temptation to light that cigarette, assure and console yourself by saying "these cravings will soon be a thing of the past" and also try your best to wait until the cravings are no longer there. It can be of immense help to have strategies to cope with those urge by preparing before that that comes.

Try to distract yourself

Clean the plates you've eaten from, watch an educative video, take a warm bath, also you can call a friend. You can engage in any activity, it does not matter the ones you embark on, what you're looking to achieve here is keeping your mind away from smoking.

Bring to your remembrance the reasons you decide to stop the habit:

Take note or put your focus on the reasons you want to stop the habit of smoking, also remind yourself or look at it from the health benefits you're going to derive from quitting this habit. Those health benefits are;

Your risk of getting disease of the heart will be reduced.

Your risk of having cancer of the lung will be reduced.

You will not be sounding like you swallow a frog when talking.

Other general benefits are: you'll appear very elegant; you'll save a lot of money. When I was into this habit I used to spend money on buying cigarette for myself and my friends, I was not able to save money, every money that gets into my hand is going straight to cigarette but when I stopped, they was immense change in how I save money. I was able to save a lot. So saving money is one of the benefit of quitting this money consuming habit, also another benefit you get from quitting is your self-esteem and confidence will be intact and enhanced; back then one of my friend who smoke, says that his reasons for smoking is to gain more confidence, but he usually complain that even though he indulge in this act to gain confidence, his confidence keep going down the drain. So I gave him all these tips and he was able to quit in no time and now his self-esteem and confidence is on a higher level, quitting this habit will help to give you confidence.

You should not put yourself in a tempting scenario:

The things you do or a place you visit can make you want to smoke. When this happen, leaving that place or stopping what you're doing can play a key role in helping you. If the place you visit will give you the urge to smoke, you should not visit that place, stay far away from there, staying there will tempt you to smoke a cigarettes.

Those places you visit that can trigger your cravings are:

Restaurant where they are smoking cigarette

In a friend's house who is a chain smoker

In a bar or brothel etc. So if you really want to quit this habit don't visit all these places that smoking of cigarette go on.

Give yourself gift:

Celebrate the goals you're able to achieve and make provision to continue. Gift yourself whenever you say no and defeat those things that will push you to smoke this will help in motivating you to press on. You can gift yourself a cake, chocolate, watching your favorite show, cooking and eating your favorite food etc.

Chapter 19: Organic And Also Holistic Solutions

Among the greatest troubles individuals have with cigarette smoking cessation is to obtain the tar as well as pure nicotine from their systems, in addition to all the various other poisonous substances that remain to make one long for those awful cigarettes.

Make a strategy.

Numerous individuals just do not understand exactly how to unwind and also require to find out methods, various other compared to smoking cigarettes. Yoga exercise as well as reflection are couple of fantastic means of relaxing.

By proceeding to compensate on your own you'll additionally recognize why you have brand-new factor to really feel pleased of on your own as well as your self-worth will certainly expand; this in turn will certainly aid with those unfavorable feelings you're attempting to regulate.

We've pointed out some organic manner ins which one can do this by yourself, however exactly what regarding organic herbs or holistic treatments? Can any of these assistance, as well as if so, just how do they function to not just free your body of these contaminants, yet to motivate you to give up cigarette smoking?

And also it could appear odd, however when you're under anxiety, this is an appropriate time to obtain included with volunteer or philanthropic job. It aids to place your very own issues in viewpoint when you see just how lots of various other individuals have points a lot even worse compared to you do, as well as in enhancement, it could assist you really feel great concerning on your own and also your success.

Return to the listing you made formerly concerning where when you illuminate and also see the number of times you're smoking to soothe stress and anxiety, monotony, irritation, or any one of these various other damaging feelings. Currently think of just what you could do to obtain around these points while stopping.

Managing tension.

And also do not fret about exactly what other individuals could think about these points, such as if you intend to occupy knitting or version structure. This is for you as well as your objectives, except other individuals to authorize or .

Obtain some paper as well as a pen now and also draw up all the important things you could do to aid you make it through the moments of stress as well as monotony that are simply component of day-to-day life, which you recognize are visiting exacerbated when you quit smoking cigarettes.

Anxiety is just one of the leading forerunners to smoking cigarettes, as well as among one of the most usual factors that individuals that have actually given up smoking cigarettes return. Lots of record that they got cigarettes once more throughout points such as examinations, hurried jobs at the office, hard times in their marital relationship, and so forth.

Several holistic as well as natural solutions function by boosting your general state of mind and also overview so regarding be much better ready emotionally and also psychologically to surrender cigarettes. Several of these consist of:

Chromium is a normally taking place trace element which assists the body to damage down healthy protein and also fat. It is likewise recognized to help with the reliable usage of insulin, consequently assisting the body to keep typical blood glucose degrees and also avoid the sugar desire frequently connected with pure nicotine drawback.

While Hypericum aids to stabilize serotonin degrees in the human brain and also make sure the healthy and balanced performance of the whole nerve system, Scuttelaria works as a peripheral nervous system restorative as well as protects against the sleeping disorders and also migraines generally connected with pure nicotine drawback.

It is likewise popular that reduced blood glucose degrees (hypoglycemia) could create impatience, which could make it harder to stand up to having a cigarette.

Hypericum as well as Scuttelaria laterifolia are 2 natural herbs popular for their helpful results on state of mind as well as nerve system wellness.

Various other usual components in cigarette smoking cessation items usually motivate tranquil as well as ease uneasyness, and also normally are:

If you could obtain those toxic substances as well as poisonous substances from your system as swiftly as feasible, not just will this assist with your cigarette yearnings, it will certainly obtain you when traveling to health and wellness that considerably quicker!

Detoxifiers.

Arsenicum Cd

Caladium Seguinum

Carbolicum Acidum

Daphne Indica

Eugenia Jambosa -

Kali Phosphoricum -

Lobelia Inflata -

Nicotinum -

Nux Vomica -

Plantago Significant -

Saccharum Officinale -

Staphysagria -

Tabacum -

Thuja Occidentalis

There are several holistic as well as natural detoxifiers. A few of one of the most prominent consist of:

The reality that you're attempting to stop cigarette smoking ought to be at the top of that listing! There is a clinical basis for sensation that smoking cigarettes unwinds as well as soothes you. Several individuals merely do not understand just how to unwind and also require to discover strategies, various other compared to cigarette smoking.

And also we could likewise aid by offering our bodies the required devices it requires for this. This suggests appropriate fiber, fruit, veggies, and also water.

By staying clear of offering our bodies harmful chemicals to begin with, we could substantially help our very own systems in cleaning. This indicates staying clear of convenience food, consisting of refined types of food, deep-fried types of foods, and also junk foods, as these generally have awful ingredients.

Foeniculum vulgare (Fennel) has actually been made use of considering that old times as an all-natural hunger suppressant as well as was commonly made use of to stop 'growling tummies' throughout worship. Aside from its all-natural diuretic buildings, Fennel likewise advertises regular liver, kidney as well as spleen wellness and also serves for acidic tummies. A lot more lately, Fennel has actually been revealed to assist ease indigestion and also colic particularly.

The body has its very own systems in position for eliminating poisonous chemicals as well as various other such waste; frequently just what is required is merely some assistance in relocating this procedure along.

Organic detoxification.

There are significant advantages one could stem from dealing with the diet regimen, and also assisting with the cigarette smoking yearnings is merely among them. Whether you're interested in holistic solutions or just desire to attempt to obtain rid of these poisonous substances on your very own, there are numerous organic methods you could clean on your own of these dreadful contaminants.

Taraxacum officinalis (Dandelion) was typically made use of in Indigenous American medication and also is located in several components of the globe today. It consists of bitter concepts that have a revitalizing result on the liver as well as digestion system.

Smoking cigarettes is not simply concerning a physical food craving, basically any kind of cigarette smoker will certainly inform you that. If they're urging you to maintain on smoking cigarettes so that they do not really feel left out or do not really feel bad regarding their choice to maintain cigarette smoking, is this individual truly a good friend to you?

Pelargonium reniforme is a medical plant understood to generations of Khoi/San offspring as well as Xhosa standard therapists for its health-promoting buildings. Understood as 'Umckaloabo', it is generally utilized for an array of healing features as well as is well understood for its helpful ability on liver operating and also as a digestive system restorative.

Nux Vomica aids promote guts.

Bryonia Alba supplies general digestive system assistance.

Lycopodium Clavatum assists the lymphatic system.

Fumaria Officinalis avoids poisoning as well as cleanses blood.

Calcarea Phosphorica assists keep a well balanced metabolic rate.

Natrum Sulphuricum boosts the constitution and also water retention.

Berberis Vulgaris promotes the kidneys as well as gallbladder.

Colocynthis promotes the body's organic procedure of removal of contaminants, both inside and also on the surface.

Prior to you diminish to the drug store or make a visit with your medical professional, you succeed to evaluate the adhering to details concerning each of these alternatives to make sure that you could be a lot better prepared making the ideal option for you.

Chapter 20: 10 Things To Stop Doing When You Quit Smoking

We all want this quit to be the quit—the one that lasts us a lifetime. We're looking for permanent freedom from nicotine addiction when we stub out the last cigarette, signaling the beginning of smoking cessation—even though most of us doubt our ability to succeed in the long-term.

With some education about what to expect when we quit smoking and a few tools to help us along, we can all find the freedom we dream so much of, a life that no longer includes thoughts of smoking or the smallest twinge of desire for a cigarette.

Misconceptions about the nature of nicotine addiction and the process of

Quitting tobacco can set smokers who are trying to quit up for failure. Build a strong quit program by educating yourself about what to expect when you stop smoking.

Learning about common pitfalls puts you in the best position to avoid them and finally become smoke-free.

1. Don't Be Impatient

It is a natural tendency to quit smoking and expect to be over it within a month. That would be nice (very nice!), but it doesn't work that way.

When we quit smoking, we're letting go of a habit that most of us have carried for many years, if not all of our adult lives. It's only fair to expect that breaking down the old associations that tied us to smoking and replacing them with new, healthier habits will take some time.

Remember, smoking cessation is a process, not an event.

Sit back, relax, and think of time as one of your best quit buddies. The more time you put between you and that last cigarette you smoked, the stronger you'll become. Have patience with yourself, and with the process.

2. Don't Worry About the Future

Nicotine withdrawal plays mind games with us early on in smoking cessation. We think about smoking all of the time, and we worry that we'll always miss our cigarettes. It's called "junkie thinking," and we all go through a certain amount of it as we recover from nicotine addiction.

For the new Quitter, it can be paralyzing to think about never lighting another cigarette. Thoughts like this, if left unchecked, can easily lead to a smoking relapse.

If you find yourself feeling panicked about your smoke-free future, pull out of it by focusing your attention only on the day you have in front of you. It takes practice and patience to stay in the here and now, but it can be done, and it is a great way to maintain control over your Quit program.

It is the truth that today is where your power to affect change in your life is, and always will be. You can't do a thing about what happened yesterday, or about what is yet to come tomorrow, but you sure can control today.

We all spend so much time living in the past or the future, while the present moments of today go by unnoticed. The next time your mind wanders ahead or back, consciously pull yourself out of it by narrowing your attention to the moments you're living right now.

3. Don't Be Negative

It's been said that the average person has approximately 66,000 thoughts on any given day and that two-thirds of them are negative. It will probably come as no surprise that we aim many of those negative thoughts directly at ourselves. Face it, we're almost always our own worst critics.

Start paying attention to your thoughts, and banish those that don't serve your best interests. Be kind to yourself and stop lamenting the things you can't change, such as the years you spent smoking.

Look at past quit attempts not as failures, but as experiences you can learn from. Think about all of the positive changes you're creating in your life by quitting tobacco now and remember to use the value of today to your advantage.

Successful long-term cessation always starts with our thoughts.

Keep your eyes on the prize and develop an attitude of gratitude. We have a way of believing what we tell ourselves over and over, so don't feed yourself negatives. Affirm the changes you are working to create in your life, and action will follow more easily.

4. Don't Neglect Yourself

Early smoking cessation is a time when you should be taking extra care to make sure all of your physical needs are met. The following list of tips will help you weather nicotine withdrawal more comfortably:

• Eat a well-balanced diet: Your body needs good quality fuel now as it works to flush the toxins from cigarettes out of your system.

• Get more rest: Chances are, nicotine withdrawal will leave you feeling fatigued for a few weeks. If you're tired, don't fight it. Sleep more if you can.

• Drink water: Water is a great quit aid. It helps you detox more quickly, works well as a craving-buster, and by keeping yourself hydrated, you'll feel better overall.

• Exercise daily: Exercise benefits both physical and mental health, and it's another good way to manage cravings to smoke. Walking is a low-impact aerobic workout that is a good choice for those of us leading inactive lives. Be sure to check in with your doctor before starting a new exercise regimen.

• Take a daily multi-vitamin: Cigarettes deplete our bodies of many nutrients, so give yourself the boost that a good multi-vitamin provides for the first few months of smoking cessation. It may help you regain your energy more quickly.

Taking care of your body, especially as you move through early cessation, will help you minimize the discomforts of nicotine withdrawal.

Remember, while nicotine withdrawal may not be a pain-free experience, it is a temporary phase of recovery that we all have to go through to get through.

5. Don't Drink Alcohol

Alcohol and tobacco go hand-in-hand. New quitters are tender. Putting yourself into a social setting where you're tempted to drink alcohol too soon after quitting can be dangerous. Don't rush it. The time will come when you can have a drink without it triggering the urge to smoke, but don't expect that to be within the first month, or perhaps even the first few months.

We're all a little different in how we move through the process of kicking nicotine addiction, so relax any preconceived notions you might have about how long recovery should take. Instead, focus on your own situation.

If there is an engagement coming up that involves alcohol and you feel nervous about that, take it as a signal to proceed with caution. Consider postponing until you're feeling stronger. And if that's not an option, work out a plan ahead of time for how you'll manage the event smoke-free.

It's no exaggeration that you are working hard to save your life by quitting smoking, so give cessation the attention it deserves.

Keep your quit program in the top slot of your list of priorities for as long as it takes. You should do whatever you need to do to maintain your "sobriety."

6. Don't Overdo It

We've talked about taking care not to neglect our physical health while going through nicotine withdrawal, but our emotional well-being is every bit as important. Stress and anger are probably two of the biggest smoking triggers we face, and they can build up and threaten our quit programs if we're not careful.

Early cessation creates its own tension, and that can be overwhelming when paired with the stresses of daily life if you let it be. Don't let yourself get run down to the point of exhaustion, and take time every single day to relieve stress with an activity that you enjoy.

Whether it's time alone with a good book, a hot bath, or working on a hobby, think of this as insurance for your quit program, not as time spent selfishly.

When you're well-rested and calm, you are much better equipped to meet the daily challenges smoking cessation presents, so spoil yourself a little each day.

7. Don't Take Yourself Too Seriously

You will have bad days. Expect and accept that. Such is smoking cessation, and such is life. On those off days, vow to put yourself in "ignore mode." In other words, don't focus on the negative atmosphere of your thoughts.

Instead, do what you can to distract and ignore your bad mood. Sometimes the best thing we can do is get out of our own way. Our minds can make small issues big and create drama out of every little thing when our moods are out of whack.

When you have a bad day, use it as an excuse to pamper yourself a little. If all else fails, call it a day earlier than usual and go to bed.

Nine times out of ten you'll wake up feeling 100% better the next day, and when you do, you'll be grateful to still be smoke-free.

8. Don't Hesitate to Ask for Help

Statistics show that people who quit smoking with a healthy support system in place have a much higher rate of long-term success with smoking cessation. In addition to the support, you might receive from friends and family, consider adding some online support to your quit program. The smoking cessation forum here offers some of the best support the Internet has to offer.

9. Don't Think You Can Smoke Just One Cigarette

Many a good quit program has been lost to thoughts of being able to control our smoking habits. Don't fall for it. The only way to keep the beast at bay is to keep nicotine out of your system.

If you decide to go ahead and smoke just one cigarette, or for just one night, chances are you'll be back to the slavery that nicotine addiction is in short order. You may even find yourself smoking more than you used to.

When it comes to smoking cessation, there is no such thing as just one cigarette. They travel in packs.

Just as success with smoking cessation begins in the mind, so does a smoking relapse. Always. If unhealthy thoughts of smoking come up, and you can't shake them, it's time to renew your resolve.

10. Don't Forget Why You Wanted to Quit

You quit smoking for a reason. Probably several. Don't let time and distance from the habit cloud your thinking. Keep your memory green by reviewing your reasons for quitting often.5 They will never be less true as time goes by, but they can feel less urgent if you're not careful.

Smoking cessation is a journey. Take it one simple day at a time, and you'll find that what started out as a difficult task soon enough becomes an enjoyable challenge.

Chapter 21: Smoking Does Not Relieve Stress Or Provide Relaxation

"With the new day comes new strength and new thoughts." Eleanor Roosevelt

May be you keep smoking because you think it relaxes you. But, as you might already know, nicotine is a stimulant—a category of drugs that is opposite of relaxation. Smoking does not "calm your nerves" or relax you. Rather, cigarette raises your blood pressure and heart rate. The nicotine kick is quick. And that is the primary reason why nicotine is such an effective addiction mechanism. Nicotine also leaves the body quickly, which prompts further urges to get more of it. And you smoke more to get more nicotine, which prompts further urges, and the cycle continues. Once you accept what smoking and nicotine is doing to you, you can come to an understanding that the only stress that a cigarette is relieving is the stress that is generated from the urge for the lack of nicotine.

If smoking actually relieves external stress and achieves relaxation, smokers would be the most relaxed and stress-free people in the world. But do you think that is true or even plausible? The opposite is true. Smokers are some of the most stressed out and agitated people. Once you accept your nicotine addiction, the reason for the smoker's irritability and tenseness is obvious. Once the effects of nicotine wears off—which is quick—the smoker has the urges to smoke more. And when a smoker cannot have another smoke for the time being, that creates the stress. The stress for more nicotine. There may be many occasions to bring about such a stress. Indeed, smokers spend most of their lives in places where they cannot smoke. May be you are at a park that does not allow smoking. Or you are at work waiting for that "smoke break." Or you are in a restaurant, which undoubtedly is non-smoking in these days. Or you are in an airplane. Or you are with family who does not want you to smoke (or does not know that you smoke). Smokers in these situations are tense, in a sense of panic, and often cannot think of anything other than to scope out the next opportunity to feed their addiction. And imagine the panic that smokers feel when they are out of cigarettes late at night and "need" to smoke. Nonsmokers do not have to feel this panic or stress. Realize that it is the cigarette itself that creates and perpetuates the stress. By having a cigarette, you are guaranteeing to have the stress of worrying about the next smoking opportunity. Your addiction to cigarette adds stress to an otherwise pleasant walk in the park, and exacerbates your stress levels in situations that are already stressful, such as an important meeting.

And what happens when you light that cancer stick in your mouth? If you were like me, you would immediately regret lighting it up and ask yourself "Why am I smoking?" Cigarette addiction is in a way unlike many other addictions. Cigarette is desirable only when you cannot have it, and it immediately ceases being desirable the moment you actually taste it. Lighting that cigarette merely relieves the tension that was created by the last nicotine stick that you have sucked on. It merely feeds the nicotine beggar inside you, but just for a little while, and the vicious cycle continues with your next cigarette, and on and on. Smokers often confuse the relief they get from a cigarette. Smoking does not relieve any stress that is not caused by the cigarette itself. For example, the stress that you might have had from that big meeting you have in an hour is still there, if not exacerbated by the rise in blood pressure resulting from the nicotine. At the same time, smoking generates the urges for more nicotine in the future, causing further stressful situations to come in the near future. Indeed, some people try to pre-empt such situations by becoming chain smokers. Chain smokers are some of the most stress-ridden people in the world. And make no mistake about it: smoking is contributing to the stress—and likely the primary cause of stress—in chain smokers.

Some smokers have also created a rationalization in their mind that smoking helps them concentrate. This is merely another mind trick conjured up by the nicotine beggar inside them. Smoking cannot provide you with better concentration for the same reason that it does not relieve stress. It is indeed difficult to concentrate better when you have to mind the cigarette beggar begging you to feed it more nicotine. Nonsmokers do not need to worry about such things. And think about the act of smoking. First, you often have to go out of your way to find a place where you can smoke and hold a burning object in your hand for several minutes at a time many times a day, interrupting whatever you were doing. Smoking is nothing but a distraction to whatever you want to concentrate on.

Aside from the stress created by the nicotine addiction, there may be stress that is caused by external circumstances resulting from cigarette smoking. Smoking in public places—like restaurants, bars, workplaces, and parks—are becoming less and less common, due in part to cities and other government entities passing laws prohibiting smoking in certain places. This is also due in part to decades of public education that has rightfully informed the public that smoking is harmful not only to the smoker but also to everyone around the smoker, due to secondhand smoke. While smoking may have been widely accepted socially in the distant past, those days are long gone. Smoking is undoubtedly an antisocial activity in the modern world. Have you ever been on the receiving end of those disapproving eyes from friends or strangers when you took out a cigarette to smoke in a public place? This happens even in places where smoking is not prohibited. But who can blame them—you are putting nonsmoker's health at risk through secondhand smoke coming from your cigarette.

Stress can come also from the fact that you have friends, family, or loved ones that want you to quit smoking. If you are like me, you may have even promised your spouse or significant other that you will not smoke. And I am ashamed to admit that countless times I have broken that promise. Sometimes I have tried to hide from my wife the fact that I have smoked, by smoking in secret, and then brushing my teeth and washing my hands. That tactic has never really worked, as my wife has a nose like a bloodhound, and it is difficult to wipe clean the nasty cigarette smell in your mouth, tongue, fingers, and hair. I have always dreaded disappointing my wife that I have broken my promise to stop smoking. But even in the face of such a stress, I had often given in to my addiction and acted to feed the nicotine beggar inside me. I felt like a fraud and a criminal, smoking in secret from my wife, afraid whether she would find out that I smoked, afraid that she would find the cigarettes I had hidden in the garage. Nonsmokers do not have to worry about whether others can smell the rotten cigarette on you or whether others can see the black and brown stains on your teeth. Nonsmokers similarly do not have to worry about all the complications in interpersonal relationships that arise because of your vile addiction to nicotine.

Such is the nature of cigarette addiction—it causes stress inside you through your physical and mental addiction to the substance, and it causes stress externally through your personal relationships and with the public at large. The notion that a cigarette "relaxes" you is a myth created by a smoker's mind to rationalize the nicotine addiction. Do not fall for this mind trick.

Chapter 22: Five Ways To Quit Smoking

Deciding that you are now ready to quit smoking is only half the battle. Knowing where to start on your path to becoming smoke-free can help you to take the leap. We have put together some effective ways for you to stop smoking today.

Tobacco use and exposure to second-hand smoke are responsible for more than 480,000 deaths each year in the United States, according to the American Lung Association.

Most people are aware of the numerous health risks that arise from cigarette smoking and yet, "tobacco use continues to be the leading cause of preventable death and disease" in the U.S.

Quitting smoking is not a single event that happens on one day; it is a journey. By quitting, you will improve your health and the quality and duration of your life, as well as the lives of those around you.

To quit smoking, you not only need to alter your behavior and cope with the withdrawal symptoms experienced from cutting out nicotine, but you also need to find other ways to manage your moods.

With the right game plan, you can break free from nicotine addiction and kick the habit for good. Here are five ways to tackle smoking cessation.

1. Prepare for quit day

Once you have decided to stop smoking, you are ready to set a quit date. Pick a day that is not too far in the future (so that you do not change your mind), but which gives you enough time to prepare.

There are several ways to stop smoking, but ultimately, you need to decide whether you are going to:

• Quit abruptly, or continue smoking right up until your quit date and then stop

• quit gradually, or reduce your cigarette intake slowly until your quit date and then stop

Research that compared abrupt quitting with reducing smoking found that neither produced superior quit rates over the other, so choose the method that best suits you.

Here are some tips recommended by the American Cancer Society to help you prepare for your quit date:

• Tell friends, family, and co-workers about your quit date.

• Throw away all cigarettes and ashtrays.

• Decide whether you are going to go "cold turkey" or use nicotine replacement therapy (NRT) or other medicines.

• If you plan to attend a stop-smoking group, sign up now.

• Stock up on oral substitutes, such as hard candy, sugarless gum, carrot sticks, coffee stirrers, straws, and toothpicks.

• Set up a support system, such as a family member that has successfully quit and is happy to help you.

• Ask friends and family who smoke to not smoke around you.

• If you have tried to quit before, think about what worked and what did not.

Daily activities – such as getting up in the morning, finishing a meal, and taking a coffee break – can often trigger your urge to smoke a cigarette. But breaking the association between the trigger and smoking is a good way to help you to fight the urge to smoke.

On your quit day:

- Do not smoke at all.

- Stay busy.

- Begin use of your NRT if you have chosen to use one.

- Attend a stop-smoking group or follow a self-help plan.

- Drink more water and juice.

- Drink less or no alcohol.

- Avoid individuals who are smoking.

• Avoid situations wherein you have a strong urge to smoke.

You will almost certainly feel the urge to smoke many times during your quit day, but it will pass. The following actions may help you to battle the urge to smoke:

• Delay until the craving passes. The urge to smoke often comes and goes within 3 to 5 minutes.

• Deep breathe. Breathe in slowly through your nose for a count of three and exhale through your mouth for a count of three. Visualize your lungs filling with fresh air.

• Drink water sip by sip to beat the craving.

• Do something else to distract yourself. Perhaps go for a walk.

Remembering the four Ds can often help you to move beyond your urge to light up.

2. Use NRTs

Going cold turkey, or quitting smoking without the help of NRT, medication, or therapy, is a popular way to give up smoking. However, only around 6 percent of these quit attempts are successful. It is easy to underestimate how powerful nicotine dependence really is.

NRT can reduce the cravings and withdrawal symptoms you experience that may hinder your attempt to give up smoking. NRTs are designed to wean your body off cigarettes and supply you with a controlled dose of nicotine while sparing you from exposure to other chemicals found in tobacco.

The U.S Food and Drug Administration (FDA) have approved five types of NRT:

- Skin patches

- Chewing gum

- Lozenges

- Nasal spray (prescription only)

- Inhaler (prescription only)

If you have decided to go down the NRT route, discuss your dose with a healthcare professional before you quit smoking. Remember that while you will be more likely to quit smoking using NRT, the goal is to end your addiction to nicotine altogether, and not just to quit tobacco.

Contact your healthcare professional if you experience dizziness, weakness, nausea, vomiting, fast or irregular heartbeat, mouth problems, or skin swelling while using these products.

Conclusion

Quitting the habit of smoking can be very hard and difficult but like other addiction with persistent and focus to quit you'll surely achieve your goal. So get the book and go through it, try and practice any information you see in this book and I assure you within a short period of time you'll not even remember whether if weed or cigarette exist

www.ingramcontent.com/pod-product-compliance
Lightning Source LLC
Chambersburg PA
CBHW071830080526
44589CB00012B/970